Niemann-Pick Disease

UNI-MED

UNI-MED Verlag AG
Bremen - London - Boston

Mengel, Eugen:
Niemann-Pick disease/Eugen Mengel.-
1st edition - Bremen: UNI-MED, 2022
(UNI-MED SCIENCE)
ISBN 978-3-8374-2444-7

Printed in Europe

MEDICINE - STATE OF THE ART

UNI-MED Verlag AG, one of the leading medical publishing companies in Germany, presents its highly successful series of scientific textbooks, covering all medical subjects. The authors are specialists in their fields and present the topics precisely, comprehensively, and with the facility of quick reference in mind. The books will be most useful for all doctors who wish to keep up to date with the latest developments in medicine.

Preface

It's been a few years since I visited Seville and especially the magnificent Casa de Pilatos from the 15th century in the old city center. The building represents a wonderful synthesis of Moorish and Spanish cultures. A Janus head can be found in the inner courtyard. The two faces look curiously, but also a little fearfully, in opposite directions. Niemann-Pick disease spontaneously came to my mind. The sculpture seems to be of one person, but the two faces represent two different identities. This is the exact association I have with Niemann-Pick disease. We have to distinguish the sphingomyelinase deficiency, Niemann-Pick disease type A & B, from the intracellular lipid transport defect, Niemann-Pick disease type C. This book presents these two entities as genetically and molecular-biologically distinct diseases, and for that reason, they will be discussed seperately in the following. The fact that the Janus faces look in opposite directions is a meaningful symbol that the different biology of the diseases also requires different therapeutic approaches. While the sphingomyelinase deficiency suggests the therapeutic principle of enzyme replacement, therapeutic substrate reduction must be considered in Niemann-Pick type C.

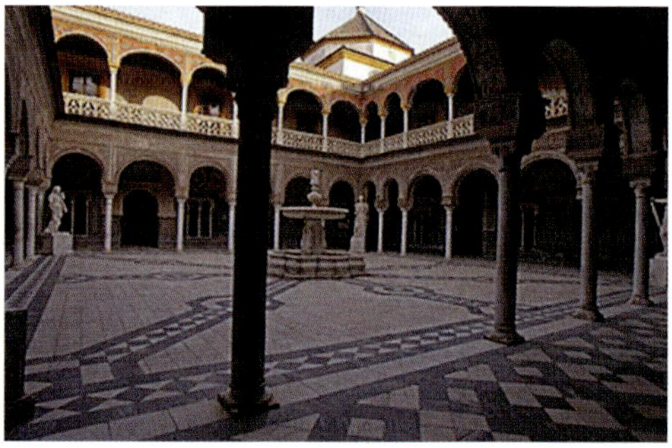

Families and patients, as well as their physicians, often ask me for an English-language edition of our book on Niemann-Pick disease. New findings in the field of basic research, a better understanding of clinical features, improved diagnostic options – especially to differentiate more easily between Niemann-Pick type C and sphingomyelinase deficiency (Niemann-Pick type A & B) –, and specific new therapeutic approaches are further arguments for creating such an edition. Prof. Michael Beck and I had already revised and updated the previous chapters for the second German-language edition that has just been published. At the suggestion of colleagues, we have added an additional chapter on "Diagnosis". This chapter in particular can be used as a quick reference work. The chapter shows which clinical symptoms corroborate a suspected diagnosis and how the diagnosis is confirmed in the laboratory.

This edition is especially dedicated to all patients with a Niemann-Pick disease and the active Niemann-Pick advocacy group.

This edition could be realized with the support of the company Gen-Orph. Thank you very much!

Hochheim, December 2021 *Eugen Mengel*

In addition, I dedicate this book to my chief, teacher, advisor, colleague, role model, comrade-in-arms, and friend Professor Michael Beck, who passed away too soon in September 2022.

Foreword

Eugen Mengel did his studies of medicine at Phillipps-University, Marburg, and Goethe-University in Frankfurt from October 1986 to September 1992. Since 1994, the medical practice has been conducted in the pediatric setting with infants, toddlers, school-age children, and adolescents and adults in some trials.

In 1994 Eugen Mengel joined the lysosomal storage disorders group named Villa metabolica of Michael Beck UMC Mainz. He was the responsible consultant for Gaucher and Niemann-Pick outpatient clinic since 1999 and later on Pompe. From 2001 to 2019 he assisted as consultant in pediatric inborn errors of metabolism in the Children´s Hospital, University of Mainz (Germany).

As sub investigator and deputy of Michael Beck he has worked on international multicenter trials for ERT in Fabry disease, Mannosidosis, Pompe disease, MPS II, MPS VI and MPS I and assisted the outpatient clinic for general metabolic, MPS, Gaucher, Niemann-Pick and Fabry patients. As principal investigator he has acted in international trials concerning NPC, ASMD, Pompe disease, Gaucher disease, LALD, Mannosidosis and Morquio disease. He has worked on biochemical diagnostic LSD laboratory from the beginning with extensive knowledge in the clinical and biochemical diagnostics of LSDs. In 2001 he received the certification for Investigator in clinical trials: KKSin Johannes-Gutenberg-Mainz. Since 2002 continuous activity as Principle Investigator in more than 25 studies according to AMG in the field of lysosomal diseases.

He has participated on student's education in pediatric hematological, oncological and metabolic diseases and given lectures about sphingolipidosis and MPS for students of medicine in biochemistry. He has been a colossal teacher, with a passionate love for medicine, metabolic diseases, and great affection for his students. One of its great virtues is his ability to synthesize and structure the most complicated ideas, concepts, and mechanisms. He makes what is difficult easy. He is a great communicator and a great teacher.

He is an active member of the SSIEM, ESGLD and EWGGD and also Board Member of several company Registries in Pompe disease (Sanofi Genzyme), Gaucher disease (Sanofi Genzyme) and Niemann-Pick type C (Actelion). As for the human side, he is an excellent person, of good character, kind and always willing to collaborate. His renowned reputation as a physician dedicated to metabolic diseases is adorned by his human qualities.

Since 2019 he is the Principle investigator, founder and CEO of the SphinCS GmbH & SphinCS Lyso non-profit UG, independed institute of clinical science in LSDs.

Barcelona, June 2022 *Mercedes Pineda*

Authors

Prof. Dr. Michael Beck †
SphinCS - Clinical Science for LSD
Geheimrat-Hummel-Platz 2
65239 Hochheim, Germany

Chapters 1., 3.

Prof. Dr. Klaus Harzer
Universitätsklinik für Kinder- und Jugendmedizin Tübingen
Neurometabolisches Labor
Hoppe-Seyler-Str. 1
72076 Tübingen, Germany

Chapter 2.

Prof. Dr. Thorsten Marquardt
Universitätsklinikum Münster
Klinik für Kinder- und Jugendmedizin
Albert-Schweitzer-Campus 1
48149 Münster, German

Chapter 4.2.2.

Dr. Eugen Mengel
SphinCS - Clinical Science for LSD
Geheimrat-Hummel-Platz 2
65239 Hochheim, German

Chapters 1., 2., 4., 5.

Dr. Janine Reunert
Universitätsklinikum Münster
Klinik für Kinder- und Jugendmedizin
Albert-Schweitzer-Campus 1
48149 Münster, German

Chapter 4.2.2.

Dr. Heiko Runz
Medical Director, Genetics at Biogen
Cambridge, Massachusetts, USA

Chapter 3.

Contents

Historical aspects of Niemann-Pick disease

1. Historical aspects of Niemann-Pick disease

In 1914 a publication titled *An unknown disease* (Niemann 1914) appeared in the 79th volume of the German pediatric yearbook "*Jahrbuch Kinderheilkunde*". The author of this article, Dr. Albert Niemann, a pediatrician from Berlin, described the case of a child of Jewish descent with an exceptionally large liver and spleen who died at the age of 18 months after rapid cerebral deterioration. An autopsy showed that liver, spleen and other organs appeared strikingly yellow in color; the histology showed large, lipid-laden cells, similar to those found in Gaucher disease. For various reasons, however, Niemann suspected a different disease in this case. On the one hand, the first symptoms appeared at a very early age and the course of disease was unusually rapid. On the other hand, the microscopic appearance of the storage cells differed from Gaucher cells.

Albert Niemann died in 1921 at the age of only 41, which is why he was called "the Unfinished" by his pediatric colleagues. He was the son of the famous opera singer (tenor) and Wagner interpreter, Albert Wilhelm Carl Niemann (1831-1917), and an actress. He completed his medical studies at the universities of Berlin, Freiburg and Strasbourg, where he also received his doctorate degree. From 1908 to 1918 he worked at the University of Berlin Children's Clinic under the direction of Prof. Cerzney. Niemann particularly devoted himself to infant medicine. In 1919, he became the medical director of a nursery in Berlin-Halensee, and in that year he was appointed associate professor of pediatrics. His book "Compendium of Pediatrics with Special Consideration of Infant Diseases" received a lot of attention.

A few years later, even before Albert Niemann's death, various German and American authors described children with identical symptoms and the same clinical course (Knox et al. 1916, Siegmund 1921). However, some of these cases were incorrectly assigned to Gaucher disease. Ludwig Pick, a German pathologist of Jewish descent, summarized all previous reports on patients with hepatosplenomegaly, combined with a rapidly progressing loss of cerebral functions, in a review and distinguished these cases, which he described as *lipoid cell splenohepatomegaly*, from Gaucher disease, mainly due to the morphological findings. Due to his creativity and scientific authority the cases of Knox and colleagues as well as Siegmund were not attributed to Gaucher disease, but rather represent an independent, different metabolic disease. In Berlin, Niemann-Pick disease was diagnosed several times between 1924 and 1926 based on spleen biopsies. In 1927 Ludwig Pick first expressed the suspicion that the substrate of the storage disease is sphingomyelin, a phospholipid characterized by L.W. Thudicum in the 1880s.

However, attempts to isolate the storage substance and to identify it chemically failed. Very soon the term *Niemann-Pick disease* was largely used for lipoid cell splenohepatomegaly. Unfortunately, Ludwig Pick was murdered in the Theresienstadt concentration camp in 1944.

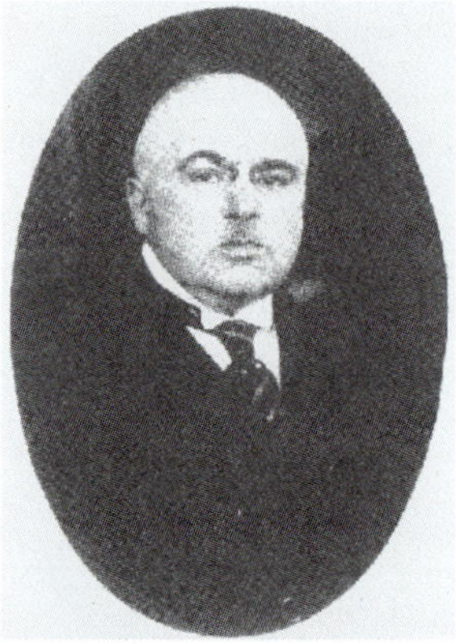

Figure 1.1: Ludwig Pick (1868-1944).

Histochemical studies showed that the storage substance was mainly composed of a phospholipid and cholesterol. The biochemist Klenk was able to identify the storage material as sphingomyelin and concluded from this that the Niemann-Pick disease could be based on a defect in an enzyme (Klenk 1934). The first adult patients were reported by Pfändler and Dusendschon in 1946 (Pfändler and Dusendschon 1946). They described two brothers who had pronounced hepatosplenomegaly, but no CNS involvement; they died at the age of 29 and 33 years, respectively.

Due to the observation of an increasing number of patients, it became apparent that Niemann-Pick

	Albert Niemann	Ludwig Pick
Born	23 February 1880 (Berlin)	31 August 1868 (Landsberg at the Warthe)
Died	22 March 1921 (Berlin)	He died completely undernourished on 3 February 1944 in the Theresienstadt concentration camp
Lineage and family	German, father famous opera singer, mother actress	The family belonged to the German-Jewish middle class, brother was a high government official
Medical field	Paediatrician	Pathologist
Study	Berlin, Freiburg and Strasbourg	Heidelberg, Leipzig, Berlin and Königsberg
Doctorate	1903 (Strasbourg)	1893 (Leipzig)
Habilitation	1918, as of 1919 appointed associate professor of pediatrics and medical director of a nursery in Berlin-Halensee	1899 habilitation in anatomical pathology, as of 1906 director of the Department of Pathological Anatomy at the Friedrichshain Clinic

Table 1.1: Biographical data of Albert Niemann and Ludwig Pick.

disease is characterized by considerable variability, both with regard to the clinical manifestation and the extent of sphingomyelin storage. Therefore, Crocker suggested dividing Niemann-Pick disease into subgroups (Crocker 1961):

- **Type A** was (and is still today) called the severe, infantile form, which is characterized by pronounced visceral and central nervous manifestation.
- Type B is characterized by severe hepatosplenomegaly in the absence of cerebral manifestation.
- Patients with both visceral and central nervous symptoms were assigned to type C, but differed from patients with type A by an overall slower and milder course.
- The designation type D (Nova Scotia variant) was reserved for patients who come from a largely isolated population group in the Canadian province of Nova Scotia. Cogan et al. observed patients who were characterized by pronounced vertical gaze palsy, ataxia and foam cells in the bone marrow. For these cases they coined the term DAF syndrome (= down gaze paresis, ataxia, foam cell), which should not be used any more.

The wide range of different symptoms observed in a large number of patients made it necessary to expand the nomenclature of Niemann-Pick disease even further to include additional subgroups: Adult patients with a visceral form of Niemann-Pick disease without cerebral involvement were called type E (Fredrickson and Sloan 1972). In 1978 Schneider et al. described two patients with a temperature-labile form of sphingomyelinase and classified them as type F (Schneider et al. 1978).

Based on today's knowledge of the etiology and pathogenesis of the various forms of Niemann-Pick disease, the terms type D, E and F are no longer used.

In 1966, Brady et al. were able to provide evidence that type A is caused by a deficiency in sphingomyelinase (Brady et al. 1966); one year later, the same enzyme defect was demonstrated in a 16-year-old patient without neurological symptoms. This proved that types A and B are only clinical variants of one and the same enzyme defect. It was soon discovered that sphingomyelinase activity is normal in patients with type C and D, and therefore this disease is an entity different from type A and B. An agreement was reached on this classification at a consensus conference in Prague in 1982 (Elleder and Jirasek 1983).

In order to better differentiate between Niemann-Pick type A, type B and type C, but also to describe the spectrum of the entity types A and B, the terminology of sphingomyelinase deficiency prevails in the more recent literature. In this context we also speak of "acid sphingomyelinase deficiency", or ASMD for short.

The molecular and genetic characterization of sphingomyelinase deficiency is closely connected with the name Edward Schuchmann. He characterized the *SMPD1* gene, produced the acid sphingomyelinase biotechnologically, bred a *SMPD1* knock-out mouse and carried out the first preclinical studies with enzyme replacement therapy, hematopoietic stem cell transplantation and gene therapy.

The pathogenesis of types C and D remained unclear for a long time. The first indications came from biochemical findings that were made on a mouse model of a lipid storage disease (*BALB/C* mouse). These animals show a reduced activity (but not a complete defect) of sphingomyelinase and some storage of sphingomyelin. The cause of the lipid storage lies in a disturbance of the esterification of exogenous cholesterol, which leads to an accumulation of free cholesterol (and to a lesser extent also of sphingomyelin and other lipids) in various tissues (Pentchev et al. 1984). Since similar histological and biochemical findings were obtained in Niemann-Pick disease type C, Pentchev and colleagues carried out biochemical analyses in fibroblasts from patients and were able to confirm that the esterification of cholesterol is actually reduced in these cells (Pentchev et al. 1985). The storage of free cholesterol can be detected by a specific stain (called Filipin test) in cultured fibroblasts. The Filipin test is still the first diagnostic step in diagnosing Niemann-Pick type C disease.

It soon turned out that Niemann-Pick disease type C does not have a uniform genetic cause: Steinberg and colleagues brought fibroblasts from two different patients together in culture and found that the Filipin staining became negative in some combinations of cells, suggesting that the biochemical defect could be corrected (Steinberg et al. 1994). As a consequence of these studies, two complementation groups could be defined, which are designated as Niemann-Pick type C1 and type C2. In 1997 the gene responsible for Niemann-Pick C1 was identified. It is located on the long arm of chromosome 18 (18q11-q12; Carstea et al. 1997). The product of the *NPC1* gene is a large glycoprotein containing 1,252 amino acids that is bound to membranes (Higgins et al. 1999).

Naureckiene and colleagues were able to isolate a lysosomal protein called HE1 which can be detected in high concentrations in testicular tissue and which has the ability to bind cholesterol. Since this protein is expressed in a large number of tissues, it has been suggested that, in addition to its role in sperm maturation, it has more extensive functions in the organism. Due to the high binding capacity of HE1 to cholesterol, the hypothesis was put forward that it could be involved in the pathogenesis of Niemann-Pick type C. And indeed, various mutations in the gene that codes for the HE1 protein were discovered in patients with type C2 (but not with type C1) Niemann-Pick disease (Naureckiene et al. 2000). It contains 5 exons and is located on the long arm of chromosome 14 (14q24.3). In contrast to the NPC1 protein, the NPC2 protein is a small, soluble molecule that contains only 132 amino acids. Both NPC proteins interlock during the transport of cholesterol from the lysosomes to cell membranes, but their exact function is still unknown.

The two forms of Niemann-Pick type C disease (C1 and C2) show considerable clinical variability and cannot be differentiated on the basis of clinical findings. However, the majority of cases (95%) are due to a mutation in the *NPC1* gene, while mutations in the *NPC2* gene are much rarer. In the Nova Scotia variant, formerly known as type D, the G3097>T mutation of the *NPC1* gene was found to be the cause (Greer et al. 1998).

For the treatment of the Niemann-Pick disease (types A/B and C), a large number of experimental therapeutic approaches were pursued in cell cultures, animal models and also in clinical studies. Experiments on enzyme replacement therapy with recombinant sphingomyelinase were carried out in mice with Niemann-Pick type A, whereby a decrease in lipid storage could be achieved. However, this could neither influence the neurological symptoms nor extend the life span (Miranda et al. 2000b). Better results were achieved with gene therapy (Miranda et al. 2000a). The first results of clinical studies with recombinant sphingomyelinase (olipudase alfa) in patients with ASMD type B and type A/B are now available (Niemann-Pick type B and type A/B; Diaz et al. 2021, Wasserstein et al. 2015). The first results of clinical studies with recombinant sphingomyelinase (olipudase alfa) in patients with ASMD type B and type A/B are for some time available (Diaz et al. 2021, Wasserstein et al. 2015). The phase III study has been published recently (Wasserstein et al. 2022).

Patterson and Wraith et al. published the results of a study in 2007 in which the effectiveness of the substrate inhibitor Miglustat® on the course of Niemann-Pick type C was examined. Miglustat® led to a decrease in the saccade disorder and improvement of other neurological functions such as ability to walk. On the basis of these positive study results, Miglustat® was approved for the treatment of patients with Niemann-Pick type C disease (Patterson et al. 2007). It is to be expected that, in the future, further drugs will be developed for the treatment of these patients which are based on other physiological mechanisms (apoptosis inhibitors, neurosteroids, cholesterol-binding preparations, especially cyclodextrin) (Wraith et al. 2009). Other interesting substances in clinical studies are acetyl leucine and arimoclomol. The first encouraging study results are currently available for both substances from 2021 (Mengel et al. 2021, Bremova et al. 2021).

References

Brady RO, Kanfer JN, Mock MB, Fredrickson DS. 1966. The metabolism of sphingomyelin. II. Evidence of an enzymatic deficiency in Niemann-Pick diseae. Proc Natl Acad Sci U S A 55: 366-9

Bremova-Ertl T, Claassen J, Foltan T, Gascon-Bayarri J, Gissen P, Hahn A, et al. 2021. Efficacy and safety of N-acetyl-L-leucine in Niemann-Pick disease type C. J Neurol. Online ahead of print.

Carstea ED, Morris JA, Coleman KG, Loftus SK, Zhang D, et al. 1997. Niemann-Pick C1 disease gene: homology to mediators of cholesterol homeostasis. Science 277: 228-31

Crocker AC. 1961. The cerebral defect in Tay-Sachs disease and Niemann-Pick disease. J Neurochem 7: 69-80

Diaz GA, Jones SA, Scarpa M, Mengel KE, Giugliani R, Guffon N, et al. 2021. One-year results of a clinical trial of olipudase alfa enzyme replacement therapy in pediatric patients with acid sphingomyelinase deficiency. Genet Med 23: 1543-50

Elleder M, Jirasek A. 1983. Niemann-Pick Disease. Report on a symposium held in Hlava's Institute of Pathology, Charles University, Prague 2nd-3rd September, 1982. Acta Universitatis Carolinae. Medica 29: 259-67

Fredrickson D, Sloan H. 1972. Niemann-Pick Disease In Sphingomyelin Lipidoses, ed. JB Stanbury, JB Wyngaarden, DS Fredrickson. New York: MacGraw-Hill

Greer WL, Riddell DC, Gillan TL, Girouard GS, Sparrow SM, et al. 1998. The Nova Scotia (type D) form of Niemann-Pick disease is caused by a G3097—>T transversion in NPC1. Am J Hum Genet 63: 52-4

Higgins ME, Davies JP, Chen FW, Ioannou YA. 1999. Niemann-Pick C1 is a late endosome-resident protein that transiently associates with lysosomes and the trans-Golgi network. Mol Genet Metab 68: 1-13

Klenk E. 1934. Über die Natur der Phosphatide der Milz bei der Niemann-Pickschen Krankheit. [10. Mitteilung über Phosphatide.]. Hoppe-Seyler´s Zeitschrift für physiologische Chemie 229: 151-56

Knox J, Wahl W, Schmeisser A. 1916. Gaucher`s disease in infants. Bull Johns Hopkins Hosp 27: 1

Mengel E, Patterson MC, Da Riol RM, Del Toro M, Deodato F, Gautschi M, et al. 2021. Efficacy and safety of arimoclomol in Niemann-Pick disease type C: Results from a double-blind, randomised, placebo-controlled, multinational phase 2/3 trial of a novel treatment. J Inherit Metab Dis. Online ahead of print.

Miranda SR, Erlich S, Friedrich VL, Jr., Gatt S, Schuchman EH. 2000a. Hematopoietic stem cell gene therapy leads to marked visceral organ improvements and a delayed onset of neurological abnormalities in the acid sphingomyelinase deficient mouse model of Niemann-Pick disease. Gene Ther 7: 1768-76

Miranda SR, He X, Simonaro CM, Gatt S, Dagan A, et al. 2000b. Infusion of recombinant human acid sphingomyelinase into niemann-pick disease mice leads to visceral, but not neurological, correction of the pathophysiology. FASEB J 14: 1988-95

Naureckiene S, Sleat DE, Lackland H, Fensom A, Vanier MT, et al. 2000. Identification of HE1 as the second gene of Niemann-Pick C disease. Science 290: 2298-301

Niemann A. 1914. Ein unbekanntes Krankheitsbild. Jahrbuch Kinderheilkunde 79

Patterson MC, Vecchio D, Prady H, Abel L, Wraith JE. 2007. Miglustat for treatment of Niemann-Pick C disease: a randomised controlled study. Lancet Neurol 6: 765-72

Pentchev PG, Boothe AD, Kruth HS, Weintroub H, Stivers J, Brady RO. 1984. A genetic storage disorder in BALB/C mice with a metabolic block in esterification of exogenous cholesterol. J Biol Chem 259: 5784-91

Pentchev PG, Comly ME, Kruth HS, Vanier MT, Wenger DA, et al. 1985. A defect in cholesterol esterification in Niemann-Pick disease (type C) patients. Proc Natl Acad Sci U S A 82: 8247-51

Pfändler U, Dusendschon W. 1946. La Maladie de Niemann-Pick dans le Cadre des Lipoidoses. Schweiz Med Wochenschrift 1946: 1228

Pick L. 1927. Über die lipoidzellige Splenohepatomegalie Typus Niemann-Pick als Stoffwechselerkrankung. Med Klin (Munich) 23: 1483

Schneider EL, Pentchev PG, Hibbert SR, Sawitsky A, Brady RO. 1978. A new form of Niemann-Pick disease characterised by temperature-labile sphingomyelinase. J Med Genet 15: 370-4

Siegmund H. 1921. Lipoidzellhyperplasie der Milz und Splenomegalie Gaucher. Verh Dtsch Ges Pathol 18

Steinberg SJ, Ward CP, Fensom AH. 1994. Complementation studies in Niemann-Pick disease type C indicate the existence of a second group. J Med Genet 31: 317-20

Wasserstein MP, Jones SA, Soran H, Diaz GA, Lippa N, Thurberg BL, et al. 2015. Successful within-patient dose escalation of olipudase alfa in acid sphingomyelinase deficiency. Mol Genet Metab 116: 88-97

Wasserstein, M., R. Lachmann, C. Hollak, L. Arash-Kaps, A. Barbato, R. C. Gallagher, R. Giugliani, N. B. Guelbert, T. Ikezoe, O. Lidove, P. Mabe, E. Mengel, M. Scarpa, E. Senates, M. Tchan, J. Villarrubia, Y. Chen, S. Furey, B. L. Thurberg, A. Zaher and M. Kumar 2022. A randomized, placebo-controlled clinical trial evaluating olipudase alfa enzyme replacement therapy for chronic acid sphingomyelinase deficiency (ASMD) in adults: One-year results. Genet Med. 24: 1425-1436

Wraith JE, Baumgartner MR, Bembi B, Covanis A, Levade T, et al. 2009. Recommendations on the diagnosis and management of Niemann-Pick disease type C. Mol Genet Metab 98: 152-65

Biochemistry of Niemann-Pick disease

2. Biochemistry of Niemann-Pick disease

2.1. Introduction and definitions

Currently, two fundamentally different groups of Niemann-Pick disease have to be considered:

- Niemann-Pick disease of the enzyme protein defect type (defects in the *SMPD1* gene coding for acid sphingomyelinase: Niemann-Pick disease types A, B and A/B; abbreviation for this type: ASMD (acid sphingomyelinase deficiency)
- Niemann-Pick disease due to errors of transport proteins (defects in the *NPC1* or *NPC2* gene: Niemann-Pick disease types C1 and C2; abbreviated to NPC, or NPC1 and NPC2)

The differences between ASMD and NPC greatly affect the biochemical characteristics of these diseases, but the common eponym Niemann-Pick was initially created as a catch-all for their phenotypic similarities, including the biochemical ones (Crocker and Farber, 1958). The biochemical similarity mainly concerned the storage of sphingomyelin in different tissues. The proliferation of this ubiquitous phospho-sphingolipid meant that the terms Niemann-Pick disease and sphingomyelin lipidosis were used almost synonymously for a long time. In 1961, A.C. Crocker separated groups A, B and C of Niemann-Pick disease. The medical terms Niemann-Pick types A, B and C, which are still used today, go back to this. At that time, however, a type assignment using laboratory methods was not possible, so that the attributions were likely inaccurate from today's point of view. Nevertheless, based on the clinical descriptions, biochemical aberrations of the enzymes involved in the metabolism of sphingomyelin were the obvious causes of Niemann-Pick disease.

In 1966, R.O. Brady and co-workers could demonstrate that in patients with the criteria of group A according to Crocker (1961), i.e. cases in children, the activity of acid sphingomyelinase (SMPD1) – a lysosomal enzyme that breaks down sphingomyelin – was greatly reduced. The genetic cause of this deficiency was recognized and explained the sometimes extensive accumulation of sphingomyelin in patient tissues: Niemann-Pick disease type A, a "lysosomal" lipid storage disease caused by a lack of SMPD1. The measurement of the SMPD1 in other Niemann-Pick cases showed very severe to severe reductions in activity, except in children and in some adult patients with clinically undetectable brain involvement (group B according to Crocker 1961). The elucidation of the role of the *SMPD1* gene took place in stages (Quintern et al. 1989, Schuchman et al. 1992).

In a number of Niemann-Pick patients, including those with the criteria of group C according to Crocker (1961), no or no significant reduction in SMPD1 activity could be found. It was noticeable in this group of patients that sphingomyelin accumulation was mild, but additional lipids, especially cholesterol, were sometimes severely increased in tissues. In the following decades, intensive studies were devoted to this group of patients. In 1997, E.D. Carstea and 37 coworkers found a gene that was mutated in patients in this group, namely the *NPC1* gene. It was found that the gene product, a highly complex transmembrane protein consisting of 1,278 amino acids (NPC1 protein), is involved in cellular cholesterol transport, and could thus explain the accumulation of cholesterol in NPC1 disease. The protein was located in the membranes of the late endosome or lysosome and possibly of other cell compartments. However, some infantile cases with almost the same lipid biochemical phenotype as NPC1 did not have an *NPC1* mutation. Using so-called genetic complementation attempts (fusion of NPC1 cells with the cells in question in culture), the existence of at least one additional gene defect that causes the NPC phenotype was strictly required (Vanier et al. 1996). As consequence the *NPC2* gene (also called the *HE1* gene; Naureckiene et al. 2000) was identified, which codes for a cholesterol transporting protein (NPC2 protein), which is much smaller than the NPC1 protein and has no transmembrane domains. Today there are indications that NPC2 and NPC1 proteins work together in a functional chain. Among other things, this chain causes the removal of cholesterol stored in the lysosomes, primarily of exogenous origin. Extracellular LDL is internalized via receptors, transported to the late endosome and then the lysosome, where it is split into apolipoprotein and free cholesterol. Pathogenic defects in the *NPC2* gene are around 20 times rarer than those in the *NPC1* gene. Research is being carried out to identify other gene defects in cases of unexplained NPC-like diseases.

2.2. Missing or pathological products of "Niemann-Pick genes"

It has been established that pathogenic mutations of the *SMPD1* or *NPC1* or *NPC2* gene are the causes of NPC. From an immunobiochemical point of view, it would be interesting to see how the products of gene mutations (mutant proteins, if they are present in a detectable amount) behave in the presence of antibodies directed against the normal gene products. If an immunobiochemical reaction with the mutant protein occurs, this is referred to as positive cross-reactive material (CRM). There is little data on NPC, but a lack of CRM seems to be the predominant situation. When SMPD1 replacement therapy for NPC hopefully becomes a reality in the near future, the patient's CRM status may be of importance for therapy. There are data on NPC1 that show that *NPC1* gene defects result in many gradations between the absence and clear presence of CRM (Millat et al. 2001). This is probably not surprising, because if the mutation impairs the function, but nevertheless allows the biosynthesis of a mutant protein, unchanged or hardly changed immunogenic areas (epitopes) would still be present, considering the large size of the NPC1 protein. A new development would be the use of active substances (chaperones) for specific gene mutations which make mutant NPC1 protein available which is in a metabolically reasonably effective form with the aim to improve the clinical phenotype (☞ Table 2.1; Gelsthorpe et al. 2008).

2.3. Biochemical foundations of diagnosing Niemann-Pick diseases

2.3.1. Niemann-Pick disease, SMPD1-associated

For a biochemical diagnosis the determination of the activity of SMPD1 plays a central role. The classic approach to measuring activity uses the natural substrate, sphingomyelin, but in its radioactively labeled form. In the test tube, which contains patient test material, such as preparations of blood leukocytes, homogenates of cultivated skin fibroblasts, amniotic fluid cells or chorionic cells, the rate of degradation (= activity) of sphingomyelin is monitored in comparison to normal activity. In the case of SMPD1 deficiency, activity is significantly reduced, e.g. 10% of the norm or less. Residual activity close to 10% is found, for example, in Niemann-Pick type B (adult form with little or no involvement of the central nervous system) and residual activity close to 1% is found in Niemann-Pick type A (infantile form with severe neurological symptoms), but many intermediate stages of both biochemical and clinical phenotypes are possible. There is a certain inverse correlation between the severity (as well as rate of progress) of the clinical course and the residual SMPD1 activity found, but with a range of fluctuations. Cultivated skin fibroblasts can be fed with radioactively labeled sphingomyelin. The less sphingomyelin is metabolized by the living cells, the more severe is the clinical course of the disease.

For routine diagnosis using blood leukocytes (containing little SMPD1, e.g. compared to cultured skin fibroblasts), an enzyme determination method with an artificial substrate that is remotely similar to sphingomyelin has proven itself (Van Diggelen et al. 2005). This substrate has the advantages of being sensitive to a small amount of SMPD1 in the test tube and of not requiring a radioactivity laboratory. With good laboratory technology, the diagnostic specificity is the same as with the use of radioactive sphingomyelin.

2.3.2. Niemann-Pick disease, transport protein deficiency-associated (NPC1, NPC2)

The assessment of the amount of cholesterol that has accumulated in the lysosomes of specially cultivated cells plays a central role in the biochemical diagnosis of the NPC group. Fibroblasts cultivated from the patient's skin biopsies are usually used with a cholesterol reagent (filipin) prepared from certain microorganisms. The cells are first "starved" for exogenous cholesterol. Therefore the cholesterol-containing LDL is withdrawn from the culture medium. In a further phase, LDL is added again, which is increasingly absorbed into the lysosomes of the cells, where it is split into apolipoprotein and cholesterol. In the case of NPC, the cholesterol remains in the lysosomes. It can be stained using filipin, and increased amounts can be detected using a fluorescence microscope. In normal cells, most of the cholesterol is transported away from the lysosomes, and these therefore show very little filipin reactivity. This cytochemical diagnostic test (filipin test), which is dependent on fluorescence microscopy, is neither comparable in its sensitivity nor in its specificity with the enzyme test for SMPD1. Even though the test seems to be positive in about 90% of the cases of NPC, dubious test results are not all that rare. A quantification of the filipin-stained cholesterol accumulated in the lysosomes is possible (Bartz et al. 2009). However, it must be taken into account that, as a result of biological fluctuations, there may be possible overlaps of relatively low signal intensities in pathological cases with the range of signal intensities of normal controls. Even healthy, heterozygous carriers of NPC sometimes have a moderately positive filipin test result. Before the identification of the *NPC1* gene opened up alternative diagnostic access via the mutation analysis of this gene, the group led by M.T. Vanier (1992) succeeded in making the filipin test using cultured chorionic cells available to a large number of families with NPC for a reliable prenatal diagnosis under strict conditions.

More recent lipid-analytical findings on NPC seem to show additional ways of biochemical diagnosis of NPC in order to circumvent the not optimally functioning filipin test. Monocytes isolated from the patient's blood can be multiplied in culture to form macrophage-like cells and then characterized using the lipid pattern determined by mass spectroscopy. If the cells derive from NPC1 patients, they may contain more cholesterol, ceramides, glucosylceramide and other components, compared to normal controls (G. Schmitz, Regensburg, personal communication). These macrophage cultures can also be influenced by exogenous reagents (e.g. different LDL types) and, in turn, differences between NPC1 patients and controls can be determined. One difference concerns the phosphatidylglycerol, which is increased in the cultures of NPC1 and possibly cannot be sufficiently converted into bis(monoacylglycero)phosphate, which seems to be important for the lipid transport which is disturbed in NPC. However, other research groups assume that this component is already increased a priori in the late endosymal/lysosome in NPC, i.e. can be made available more or less undisturbed (Davidson et al. 2009, Figure S4).

Biomarkers, which would be very important for monitoring the course of the NPC disease or the patient's response to therapeutic attempts (☞ Chapter 2.6.), are currently beeing researched by the group around D.S. Ory (e.g. Frolov et al. 2003) in the metabolic field of the so-called side chain oxysterols (cholesterol derivatives). There is a prospect that these oxysterols (e.g. 25- and 27-hydroxycholesterol) will serve as biomarkers in the disease and can be quantified from blood samples, etc.

2.3.3. Chitotriosidase activity in plasma

The activity of chitotriosidase in plasma is a long-known marker for a number of lysosomal storage diseases which are associated with involvement of macrophages (in which the enzyme is mainly expressed without a known physiological role). In Gaucher disease there are *extreme* increases in activity; in other diseases *lower* increases in activity. In view of the difficulty of accurate clinical and biochemical diagnosis, especially in NPC patients, the often measurable moderate increase in plasma chitotriosidase usually provides indispensable additional information (Ries et al. 2006), even though approximately 7% of people do not express chitotriosidase at all.

2.3.4. Determination of oxysterols

Oxysterols (oxidation products of cholesterol) are the most established, most accessible biomarkers with the largest evidence base in the diagnosis of NPC. It has been shown that cholestane-3b,5a,6b-triol (C-triol) and 7-ketocholesterol (7-KC) can be detected at elevated levels in the plasma of patients with NPC. C-Triol is the preferred oxysterol biomarker, due to its superior specificity and sensitivity. Elevation of C-triol and 7-KC also occur in other diseases, mainly in Niemann-Pick disease type A and B and lysosomal acid lipase deficiency. Therefore, increased oxysterol values should be interpreted with caution. Longer storage of samples at room temperature can lead to auto-oxidation of cholesterol, which can cause false-positive results.

2.3.5. Determination of lyso-sphingomyelin-509 (lyso-SM-509)

Newer biomarkers could one day eclipse oxysterols. Desirable properties include increased stability, more convenient sampling methods (e.g., dried blood spot [DBS] or urine), smaller blood volumes (e.g., DBS in infants), more convenient handling, and characteristic NPC profiles that facilitate differential diagnosis when used in multi-analyte panels. Lyso-SM-509 and other lyso-sphingolipids appear to be particularly suitable. Lyso-SM-509 is increased in the plasma of patients with NPC and NPA/B compared to controls.

The increase in lyso-SM in patients with NPC is very small compared to that in patients with NPA/B. Therefore, the measurement of combinations of biomarkers, such as lyso-SM and lyso-SM-509, is suitable for the differentiation between NPC and ASMD (NPA/B).

2.3.6. Determination of bile acids

It is known that the levels of certain bile acids are elevated in patients with NPC. The preferred analytical species is 3b,5a,6b-trihydroxy-cholanoyl-glycine. The assay can be used in DBS, plasma and urine and preanalytical auto-oxidation is not a problem. In addition, 3b,5a,6b-trihydroxy-cholanoyl-glycine appears to be more specific for NPC than C-triol.

2.4. Biochemistry of Niemann-Pick diseases that is pathogenetically relevant or suspected to be significant

2.4.1. Niemann-Pick disease, SMPD1-associated

It used to be assumed that the accumulation of sphingomyelin, caused by the lack of SMPD1 activity for lysosomal sphingomyelin degradation (hydrolysis to ceramide and phosphorylcholine), was the main cause of the pathological changes in the nerve cells and/or visceral organs in ASMD. This was evident in so far as, for example, the central nervous system neurons in Niemann-Pick type A contain such high quantities of large "storage lysosomes" (storage membranes that are oversaturated with sphingomyelin, but also secondarily enriched with gangliosides) that the whole nerve cell is inflated, or "ballooned", and thus seemed doomed to their impending cell death. There is still a lot to be said for this explanation, but all in all it is probably too simple. Additional pathomechanisms are being discussed today. We know from an animal model (☞ Chapter 2.5.) that SMPD1, actually a lysosomal enzyme with an acidic pH optimum, performs very different important functions, e.g. in general membrane formation and physiology, but also on the outer cell membrane. SMPD1 gets there by secretion and hydrolyzes sphingomyelin even in the pH conditions found there. In the case of their defect, at least in the animal model, certain microdomains with sphingomyelin accumulation arise in the cell membrane, which, for example, disrupts the distribution of GPI-anchored functional proteins. In this context it is also interesting that, in the animal model (☞ Chapter 2.5.), the phospholipid mixture of the surfactant factor is pathologically enriched with sphingomyelin on cell surfaces of the bronchial mucosa, which affects its function. Therefore this could be significant also for the pathogenesis of the sometimes very pronounced lung involvement in human Nieman-Pick disease. The hydrolysis of sphingomyelin on the cell membrane by SMPD1 is also particularly important in the area of signal transduction (Smith and Schuchman 2008). The ceramide released there by SMPD1 is a central signaling molecule. If too little signal ceramide is available due to SMPD1 deficiency, a total cellular malfunction is likely to set in. Interestingly, although the lack of SMPD1 makes the cell resistant to stress-induced apoptosis (Smith and Schuchman 2008), many other important processes are disrupted. Signal defects with an "inflammatory effect" could also be the cause of liver cirrhosis, which often occurs in slowly progressing forms of Niemann-Pick (type B), because this cannot easily be explained by the storage of sphingomyelin in hepatocytes and Kupffer cells. However, sphingomyelin storage is probably also pathogenetically relevant in itself or in addition to the fact that it evidently results in "secondary" lipid storage due to a blocking effect, for example of cholesterol in the liver of patients with Niemann-Pick type B and of GM_2 and GM_3 ganglioside in the brain of patients with Niemann-Pick type A.

2.4.2. Niemann-Pick disease, transport protein deficiency-associated (NPC1, NPC2) in general

The sequential course of the pathogenesis of NPC is still not clear, despite considerable detailed knowledge (Sturley et al. 2009). Since the NPC1 protein appears to have functional effects on a number of metabolic steps, it is sometimes called a "house-keeping protein". Its defects lead to metabolic disorders or transport disorders of multiple lipids such as cholesterol, sphingomyelin, glycolipids including gangliosides as well as phosphoglycerides and others with the consequence of their accumulation in the late endosome and lysosome (which are also summarized as "acidic cell compartments"). NPC is also a lysosomal storage disease. Other biochemical changes in NPC1, so far often only detected in cell culture models or in animal models (☞ Chapter 2.5.), are e.g. the increase in sphingosine and the decrease in calcium levels in the lysosome, the loss of allopregnanolone (an indispensable neurosteroid hormone) in the nerve cells, SMPD1 activity inhibition by the lysosomal load, or the insufficient availability of Rab9 (☞ Table 2.1). Furthermore, there is a ferritin deficiency in the liver cell, an aggregation of disturbed cytoskeletal proteins (e.g. tau with reference to Alzheimer's disease) in nerve cells and axons, an increase of cystine in the lysosome, increased activity of lysosomal enzymes (e.g. cathepsin B and D) and decreased activity of peroxisomal enzymes. In addition, many other pathological changes occur, including several in the extralysosomal region. Undoubtedly only some of the changes are a direct expression of the defect in the NPC1 protein, and many of them belong to a cascade of secondary disorders. All of them together create some kind of metabolic chaos for NPCs. This chaos also includes an activation of inflammatory factors (e.g. by increasing the activity of lysosomal enzymes), so that tissue infiltration with inflammatory cells sometimes takes place or the microglia in the brain is overactivated. In addition, autophagic and apoptotic processes, as well as oxidative stress (mitochondrial dysfunction?), are set in motion.

According to a concept that has been impressively proven experimentally (Lloyd-Evans et al. 2008), the above-mentioned increase in sphingosine in the lysosome can be regarded as the primary biochemical-pathogenetic factor in NPC1. For certain reasons, it causes a drop of the lysosomal calcium level, which disrupts the cellular calcium balance via a cross-connection between the lysosome and the cytoplasm. However, such a balance is necessary for maintaining the so-called endocytic metabolic pathway, which extends into the lysosome and prevents lipids, such as cholesterol, from accumulating there. This concept assumes that sphingosine – a central component of all sphingolipids – is specifically recognized and processed by the normal NPC1 protein. It is therefore discharged from the lysosome or its predecessors (endosomes), but not in the case of NPC1. According to this concept, one or the primary function of the NPC1 protein, also known as the "transmembrane pump", driven by a proton gradient, is seen in the excretion of sphingosine and not in the accumulation of lysosomal cholesterol. On the other hand, it is argued that findings suggest a functional independence of the NPC1 protein from its cholesterol binding capacity. The author would like to add the point of view that the increased sphingosine (☞ also Davidson et al. 2009) in NPC1 may only be released from the increased amount of sphingolipids in the lysosome by the lysosomal ceramidase. In any case, the increased sphingosine is very suspicious as a pathogenetic factor.

Arguably, the long-standing hypothesis that NPC1 protein has its primary task in removing cholesterol from the lysosome is still conceivable today. Winkler and colleagues confirmed it in 2019. NPC proteins are essential for sterol and cholesterol homeostasis. They regulate the integration of sterols into the lysosomal membrane before they are distributed to other cellular membranes. Using a combination of crystallography, cryo-electron microscopy and in vivo biochemical studies on the *Saccharomyces cerevisiae* NPC system (NCR1 and NPC2), Winkler and colleagues presented a model for sterol membrane integration. Sterols, especially cholesterol, are exchanged between the hydrophobic pockets of the vacuolar NPC2 and the membrane protein NCR1. NCR1 has positioned its N-terminal domain (NTD) to deliver a sterol into a tunnel. The NTD with luminal membrane leaflets is 50 Å away. A sterol is transported through a proton relay network of charged residues by means of a proton-driven transport through the tunnel to the membrane.

It is also conceivable that the upcoming roles of cellular cholesterol transport (e.g. from the lysosome to the plasma membrane and to the endoplasmic reticulum) normally activate the NPC1 protein (i.e. switch on its function as a transmembrane pump) in such a way that it can still perform a number of additional tasks. NPC1 defects would then result in corresponding failures. If lysosomal cholesterol accumulation is a primary event in NPC, it could lead to an increase in other substances or disorders of their metabolism without the NPC1 protein being directly involved. On the other hand, if the accumulation of glycosphingolipids is a primary event, for which there are some arguments, then an inverse sequence of disorders is conceivable. Such a sequence would even better explain the observed reduction in the cholesterol load in NPC patients by treatment with miglustat (☞ Chapter 2.6.; Lachmann et al. 2004). Miglustat primarily reduces the glycosphingolipid load, but it is precisely through this effect that it could lighten the cellular storage organelles so that they can at least partially release the storage substance partner cholesterol. In this context, it is also interesting that, in NPC, the cell is actually low in cholesterol intracellularly, with the exception of its late endosomes/lysosomes, which act as a cholesterol trap. This means that cholesterol biosynthesis is not downregulated and signaling cholesterol does not reach the corresponding receptors. Furthermore, the LXR receptors (☞ Table 2.1) cannot be activated because the corresponding cholesterol metabolites are missing, which affects, for example, the excretion of cholesterol from the brain (Repa et al. 2007). Finally, too few cholesterol esters can be formed in the endoplasmic reticulum.

A defect in the NPC2 protein apparently causes a similar metabolic chaos as a defect in the NPC1 protein. This is likely to be related primarily to the functional cooperativity of NPC1 and NPC2 proteins (Sleat et al. 2004). According to a theory that has not yet been definitively proven, the NPC2 protein captures lysosomal cholesterol first and

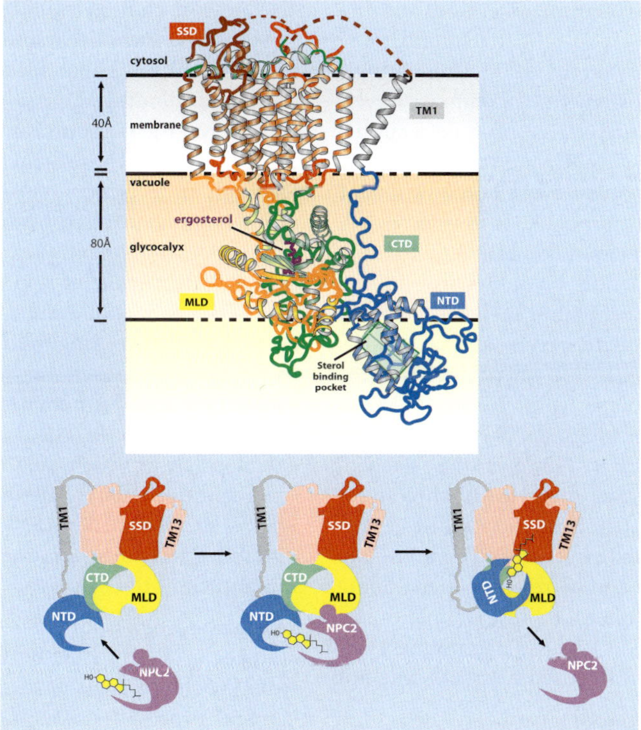

Figure 2.1: Structure of NPC1 and mechanism of cholesterol transfer (modified after Winkler et al. 2019 and Trinh et al. 2018). NPC2 transports cholesterol into the lysosome and presents the molecule to the NTD gripper of the NPC1 protein. The remainder of the NPC1 protein forms a transmembrane tunnel through which cholesterol then penetrates and can be reintegrated into membranes or made available to other cell organelles.

passes it on to the NPC1 protein. If this step does not take place due to an NPC2 defect, it is possible that downstream the intact NPC1 protein is practically inactive. Perhaps, however, a minimal function of the NPC1 protein is necessary in some organs to prevent what often occurs, for example, in NPC2 disease: lung involvement becomes so severe (with large amounts of storing macrophages) that this determines the rapid clinical course despite the simultaneous neuropathology (Bjurulf et al. 2008).

2.4.3. Niemann-Pick disease, transport protein deficiency-associated (NPC1, NPC2), central nervous system

The biochemical pathogenesis of NPC must be discussed separately for the central nervous system (CNS), because the biochemical findings in the brain of NPC patients or in the animal model differ significantly from those in visceral organs (☞ Chapter 2.5.). This is important because, as a rule, the CNS involvement determines the clinical course of the disease (there are exceptions, e.g. the predominance of lung involvement in rapidly progressing NPC2 or, very rarely, NPC1 cases without noticeable brain involvement). In contrast to visceral organs, in neuronal cells is only mild accumulation of cholesterol in NPC, and sphingomyelin, which may only accumulate as a consequence of cholesterol retention, probably is not increased. According to current view (Zervas et al. 2001), the non-severe accumulation of cholesterol in the neurons is nevertheless pathogenetically relevant and was mainly characterized in animal models (Davidson et al. 2009). But where does this increased cholesterol come from? Neurons cannot take up cholesterol through endocytosis of blood lipoproteins such as LDL. However, the astroglial cells probably provide them with cholesterol bound to apolipoprotein E for endocytotic uptake (Göritz et al. 2002), so that it can end up in the late endosome/lysosome and be retained there. Some of the neuronal cholesterol (which is functionally very important, e.g. in synapse membranes) derives from the cell's own biosynthesis and does not enter the lysosome.

In terms of lipid chemistry, the accumulation of glycosphingolipids, including gangliosides, in the nerve cells is more noticeable than the increase in cholesterol (Vanier 1999). This accumulation is considered to be very likely pathogenetically relevant (Zervas et al. 2001; Davidson et al. 2009), even if the degree of the various clinical forms of NPC can show significant individual variation. Accumulated glycosphingolipids are also found in the visceral organs in NPC, but here they are a minority compared to cholesterol and sphingomyelin. However, this is a relevant minority as it includes glycosphingolipid types such as glucosylceramide, lactosylceramide and GM_3 ganglioside as storage substances. GM_3 is the "simplest" ganglioside, the precursor of which is lactosylceramide, which itself is derived from glucosylceramide. This set of stored glycosphingolipids also occurs in the nerve cells in NPC, alongside storage substances such as GM_2 ganglioside and the metabolically related asialo-GM_2 ganglioside (in addition to less relevant glycolipid types; Vanier 1999).

The pattern of storage lipids in the nerve cells in NPC, with the apparent dominance of glycosphingolipids over cholesterol, raises the question of whether the NPC1 protein is primarily used for the discharge of cholesterol or glycolipids, especially gangliosides, from the lysosomal system. Despite the apparent molecular specificities of the NPC1 protein for binding and mediating the reaction of cholesterol, the question cannot yet be answered. The concept that the protein is equally responsible for both processes is (still) justified. A superordinate process is also possible (e.g. the "sphingosine hypothesis" mentioned in the previous section, Lloyd-Evans et al. 2008). According to new data (Davidson et al. 2009), it is conceivable that especially the GM_3 ganglioside (possibly including its precursors lactosylceramide and glucosylceramide) is processed simultaneously with the cholesterol and stored in NPC. The more complex gangliosides, of which only the GM_2 ganglioside was mentioned above, are only involved secondarily, even if they promote cholesterol storage via a different mechanism (animal model of a double mutant, Gondré-Lewis et al. 2003).

The pathogenetic potential of glycosphingolipid storage can probably also be deduced ex juvantibus from the effectiveness of miglustat therapy on the cerebral process (☞ Chapter 2.6.), because miglustat inhibits an initial step in glycosphingolipid biosynthesis and thus leads to a reduction in glycosphingolipid load for the nerve cell in NPC. Investigations on certain animal models allow the conclusion that this also indirectly reduces cholesterol storage.

When looking at the gray matter (representative of nerve cells) and the white matter (medullary substance) of the brain separately, the glycosphingolipid accumulation in NPC is mainly (but not exclusively) found in the former. In contrast, the latter shows reductions in other glycosphingolipids (galactosylceramide, sulfatide) and cholesterol (Vanier 1999) that are not related to the ganglioside series. The reduction in cholesterol, together with a certain increase in the nerve cells, seems to result in a "normal" total cholesterol content in the brain in the case of NPC. This lipid group is part of the typical lipids found in the medullary substance. Its reduction (which is very different in its degree in the various clinical forms of NPC) reflects the demyelination as a consequence of nerve cell death in the sense of a secondary leukodystrophy. In addition to the lipid changes mentioned, there are a number of other biochemical abnormalities in the NPC brain, similar to those mentioned in the previous section. Particular mention should be made of aggregations of chemically modified cytoskeletal proteins (e.g. tau protein) in the neurons and their branches, which lie parallel to the neuroaxonal dystrophy or the ectopic neurites and may be triggered by the neuronal glycosphingolipid changes (Zervas et al. 2001).

An additional pathogenetic factor appears to be significant inflammatory activity in the NPC brain. It is assumed, for example, that the microglial cells ("macrophages of the brain") are programmed towards an inflammatory reaction due to their own NPC1 defect, but are also activated by other signals (Repa et al. 2007).

2.5. Animal models

2.5.1. Niemann-Pick disease, SMPD1-associated

In 1995 (Horinouchi et al.) the acid sphingomyelinase knock out (ASMKO) mouse was created. This SMPD1–/– model has made a decisive contribution to demonstrating functions of SMPD1 that go beyond the lysosomal breakdown of sphingomyelin and include, for example, their roles in signal transduction and apoptosis. The mouse model with an age of death at approximately 8 months imitates human ASMD impressively in terms of neuropathology, visceral and other phenotypes. It has been used successfully for therapeutic studies with exogenous enzyme replacement (Miranda et al. 2000) and transfer of the human SMPD1 gene via viral vectors (Passini et al. 2005; Dodge et al. 2005; Barbon et al. 2005). As expected, when exogenous enzyme replacement with recombinant human SMPD1 (rhASM) was used, the neurological status and neuropathology were not influenced (although the visceral phenotypes were largely resolved!) because the enzyme does not overcome the blood-brain barrier. In the case of gene transfer, if it was performed by intracerebral injection, however, neuropathology and motor deficits were improved and the further death of Purkinje cells in the cerebellum (the death of which is often a "neuropathological marker" in Niemann-Pick diseases) was prevented.

The alveolar macrophages of the lungs of the SMPD1–/– mouse were a vivid model for studying the uptake of rhASM, which is used for enzyme replacement, in macrophages (Dhami and Schuchman 2004). The cells that cause most of the visceral involvement in ASMD are storage macrophages, including the alveolar macrophages of the SMPD1–/– mouse. It has been shown that the rhASM, as long as its N-linked oligosaccharides are of the "natural", complex type, is absorbed to a lesser extent by pathological macrophages than by normal ones. The uptake takes place via mannose and mannose-6-phosphate receptors, which are present in the cells of the SMPD1–/– mouse, but their activity is disturbed as an indirect consequence of the SMPD1 defect. If the oligosaccharide side chains of the rhASM were "cut" so that the mannose components were exposed, the rhASM uptake in the pathological cells increased by a factor of 10 despite the receptor disorder. This effect is important for enzyme replacement therapy in general and especially for the response in lung involvement, which is not uncommon in human ASMD, with regard to the therapy to be expected in the near future.

2.5.2. Niemann-Pick disease, transport protein deficiency-associated (NPC1, NPC2)

A large part of the findings on the "multi-factorial" pathogenesis of Niemann-Pick disease, which has already been discussed, and the therapeutic influence on individual pathogenetic factors was developed using the model of the Balb/3npc1 (NIH) mouse. This model of the NPC1 disease with a severe clinical course resulted from a spontaneous mutation and was first described in 1984. It was later characterized in more detail at the NIH and the mutation was recognized as a combination of an insertion and a deletion in the mouse equivalent of the NPC1 gene (Loftus et al. 1997). The mutation leads to a "mutilated", largely functionless NPC1 protein. There is another NPC1 mouse model as well as cat and dog models. A mouse model of NPC2 disease generated by gene targeting was also investigated (Sleat et al. 2004; Davidson et al. 2009). It was characterized as a relatively protracted NPC2 disease in mice with "hypomorphic" instead of zero expression of the NPC2 protein.

2.6. Therapeutic concepts for the possible influence of pathogenetically significant metabolic changes

2.6.1. Niemann-Pick disease, SMPD1-associated

At 24th June 2022, the European Mediciny Agency and at 31st August 2022, the U.S. Food and Drug Administration approved Olipudase alfa for intravenous infusion in pediatric and adult patients with Acid Sphingomyelinase Deficiency (ASMD), a rare genetic disease that causes premature death. Olipudase alfa is the first approved medication to treat symptoms that are not related to the central nervous system in patients with ASMD. The approval is based on studies demonstrating the safety and efficacy of olipudase alfa, with the Phase III study recently published (Wasserstein et al. 2022).

2.6.2. Niemann-Pick disease, transport protein deficiency-associated (NPC1)

Various starting points for drug therapy or other treatments of the NPC phenotype that are already applicable or may be useful in the future are shown in Table 2.1. Many results come from studies of the Balb/3npc1 (NIH) mouse, some also from (partly drug-induced) cell culture models of NPC1.

So far, intact NPC1 protein (or in rare cases NPC2 protein) cannot be supplied to the cells of the affected patient, although the defect in the protein is the root cause of the disease. In this context, Table 2.1 is intended to illustrate the following considerations: Some of the pathogenetically relevant biochemical (and other) phenotypes can evidently be influenced by active substances, so that improvements in clinical phenotypes do not seem impossible and are even partly possible through administration of miglustat. The phenotypes are based on the failure of functions that are in part metabolically close to those of the NPC1 protein and in part may also be distant from them. Primary failures probably induce secondary failures, whereby negative feedback is possible. A strategy to resolve this chaos to some extent would be to simultaneously use as many rationales from Table 2.1 as suitable for a concerted attack. For this purpose, a combination of active ingredients should be sought and optimized in such a way that the NPC patient experiences an improvement in the quality of life that justifies this kind of polypharmacy. According to the current state of knowledge, this goal does not even seem unrealistic. For example, an optimistic view in a study on the activation of the LXR receptor (☞ Table 2.1) and on the expression of certain transport proteins in NPC cells indicates that NPC1 mutations can largely be circumvented and that the function of the NPC1 protein is not the deciding factor for the circulation and excretion of cholesterol when the secondary defects in the regulation of those transport proteins are corrected by agonists or activators of the receptor (Boadu et al. 2006). The "miracle drug" CYCLO (☞ Table 2.1) reduces, among other things, the cholesterol load in the whole body and in the brain (Liu et al. 2009), particularly in the nerve cells (Davidson et al. 2009). However, the possibility of its use in humans cannot currently be assessed.

Table 2.1 is not a complete representaion. It is intended to give an idea of a range of starting points for treatment, many of which are not yet explored or have not been considered here. The author speculates that overexpression of glucosylceramide-β-glucosidase (GBA1) could have a similar effect on the NPC phenotype as overexpression of SMPD1 (third from last line of the table). Highly active GBA1 could reduce the glucosylceramide load in the nerve cells and partly in the visceral organs and thus also facilitate the efflux of cholesterol and other lipids from endosomes and lysosomes.

Substance	Function	Effect in NPC	Biochemical and/or clinical improvement (life extension) in NPC1 mouse model, or "phe-notype correction" in cell culture model	Clinical as well as neurological improvement in human NPC disease
Miglustat (Zavesca®)	inhibitor of glucosylceramide synthase	decrease in glycosphingolipid storage in the brain, second-ary influence on cholesterol increase	++	+ (human study: Patterson et al., 2009)
CYCLO (specially modified cyclodextrin, a cyclic carbohydrate)	"NPC1 protein prosthesis" with ve-hicle functions for active substances and lysosomal stor-age lipids	reduction of the storage sub-stance load in the whole body (also in the brain) as well as inflammation factors in the liver and brain, protection of endangered Purkinje cells in the cerebellum	+++	?
Arimoclomol	Amplifier of Heat Shock Protein (HSP) expression	Stimulatingcellular protein re-pair and lysosomal function	+/++	+ (human study: Mengel et al., 2021)
HP-β-Cyclodextrin i.th. Adrabetadex	"NPC1 protein prosthesis" with vehiclefunctionsfor activesubstances and lysosomal stor-age lipids	reduction of the storage sub-stance load in the whole body (also in the brain) as well as inflammation factors in the liver and brain, protection of endangered Purkinje cells in the cerebellum	+++	Final study re-sults not pub-lished, phase III study ter-minated
HP-β-Cyclodextrin intravenous	"NPC1 protein prosthesis" with vehiclefunctionsfor activesubstances and lysosomal stor-age lipids	reduction of the storage sub-stance load in the whole body (also in the brain) as well as inflammation factors in the liver and brain, protection of endangered Purkinje cells in the cerebellum	+++	Phase III study is running
Vorinostat	Histone deacety-laseinhibition	Upregulation of NPC1-, NPC2- and other proteins	+	Phase 2 and 3 trials are ex-pected
AZ-1302	Inhibition of gluco-sylceramide syn-thase (GCS) and non-lysosomal neu-tral glucosyl-ceramidase	Reduction of gangliosides and increased cytosolic glucosylceramid	+++	Phase 2 and 3 trials are ex-pected
N-Acetyl-L-Leucin	Modificatedaminoa cid	improves functional recovery and attenuates cortical cell death	+	Phase 3 trial is running

Allopregnanolone	neurosteroid, agonist for receptors (e.g. for GABA and PXR), neuroprotective, also effective in lipid exchange	improvement of the disturbed lipid trafficking, but in a time window around the 7th postnatal day of the NPC1 mouse	(+) to +	?
Oxysterols (25- and 27-hydroxy-cholesterol)	LDL-dependent sterol regulators	improvement of the disturbed lipid trafficking	+	?
LXR agonists (oxysterols and artificial ligands for the nuclear LXR receptor)	transcription factor for certain sterol transporters	increase in cholesterol excretion from the brain, decrease in neural inflammation factors, retransforming of microglia from "inflammatory" into inactive form	+	?
Curcumin (SERCA antagonist)	development of calcium levels, restitution of calcium signalling	reduction of the endosomal/lysosomal lipid load marked by intralysosomal calcium depletion (triggered by sphingosine storage?)	++	?
Glycerine, 4-phenyl-butyric acid and other chaperone proteins to be determined	reduction of misfolding of NPC1 protein, which is damaged by certain human mutations (e.g. I1061T)	higher availability of the mutated NPC1 protein, some of which is still effective like the normal variant = "defect enzyme improvement"	+	?
Tacrolimus (immunosuppressive drug) and atorvastatin (cholesterol-lowering drug)	anti-inflammatory, immunomodulatory	decrease in the inflammatory component in the brain, in combination with allogregnanolone restoration of fertility in animal models	+	?
Coenzyme Q and sesame oil (with tocopherols)	antioxidants	reducing oxidative stress?	+	?
Inhibitors of lysosomal proteases	inhibitory effects on activity	suppression of neuronal vulnerability due to overactivity of cathepsin B and D	+	?
Appendix: Effect of overexpression of the cell's own gene products				
SMPD1 overexpression	increase in sphingomyelinase activity	reduction of sphingomyelin load and thus indirectly of cholesterol load as well as other beneficial effects	+	?
Rab9 overexpression	Rab9 is a small RAS-like GTP-binding protein of the endosome that acts in shuttling cargo (substance load exchange) of the late endosome	reduction of cholesterol in the late endosome, decrease in lipid storage in neurons as well	+	?

ARF6 overexpression	ADP-ribosylation factor 6 is a small GTP-binding protein of the plasma membrane that acts in protein and lipid trafficking of the endocytotic pathway	loosening of the cholesterol blockade during substance transport out of endosomal membranes	+	?

Table 2.1: Active substances and therapeutic approaches for improving biochemical, inflammatory and clinical phenotypes in NPC1 disease. **SERCA** = sarcoplasmic/endoplasmic reticulum Ca^{2+}-ATPase.

References

Barbon CM, Ziegler RJ, Li C, Armentano D, Cherry M, Desnick RJ, Schuchman EH, Cheng SH. 2005. AAV8-mediated hepatic expression of acid sphingomyelinase corrects the metabolic defect in the visceral organs of a mouse model of Niemann-Pick disease. Mol Ther 12(3): 431-40

Bartz F, Kern L, Erz D, Zhu M, Gilbert D, Meinhof T, Wirkner U, Erfle H, Muckenthaler M, Pepperkok R, Runz H. 2009. Identification of cholesterol-regulating genes by targeted RNAi screening. Cell Metab 10(1): 63-75

Bjurulf B, Spetalen S, Erichsen A, Vanier MT, Strøm EH, Strømme P. 2008. Niemann-Pick disease type C2 presenting as fatal pulmonary alveolar lipoproteinosis: morphological findings in lung and nervous tissue. Med Sci Monit 14(8): CS71-5

Boadu E, Choi HY, Lee DW, Waddington EI, Chan T, Asztalos B, Vance JE, Chan A, Castro G, Francis GA. 2006. Correction of apolipoprotein A-I-mediated lipid efflux and high density lipoprotein particle formation in human Niemann-Pick type C disease fibroblasts. J Biol Chem 281(48): 37081-90

Brady RO, Kanfer JN, Mock MB, Fredrickson DS. 1966. The metabolism of sphingomyelin. II. Evidence of an enzymatic deficiency in Niemann-Pick diseae. Proc Natl Acad Sci U S A 55(2): 366-9

Carstea ED, Morris JA, Coleman KG, Loftus SK, Zhang D, Cummings C, Gu J, Rosenfeld MA, Pavan WJ, Krizman DB, Nagle J, Polymeropoulos MH, Sturley SL, Ioannou YA, Higgins ME, Comly M, Cooney A, Brown A, Kaneski CR, Blanchette-Mackie EJ, Dwyer NK, Neufeld EB, Chang TY, Liscum L, Strauss JF 3rd, Ohno K, Zeigler M, Carmi R, Sokol J, Markie D, O'Neill RR, van Diggelen OP, Elleder M, Patterson MC, Brady RO, Vanier MT, Pentchev PG, Tagle DA. 1997. Niemann-Pick C1 disease gene: homology to mediators of cholesterol homeostasis. Science 277(5323): 228-31

Crocker AC, Farber S. 1958. Niemann-Pick disease: a review of eighteen patients. Medicine (Baltimore) 37(1): 1-95

Crocker AC. 1961. The cerebral defect in Tay-Sachs disease and Niemann-Pick disease. J Neurochem 7: 69-80

Davidson CD, Ali NF, Micsenyi MC, Stephney G, Renault S, Dobrenis K, Ory DS, Vanier MT, Walkley SU. 2009. Chronic cyclodextrin treatment of murine Niemann-Pick C disease ameliorates neuronal cholesterol and glycosphingolipid storage and disease progression. PLoS One 4(9): e6951

Dhami R, Schuchman EH. 2004. Mannose 6-phosphate receptor-mediated uptake is defective in acid sphingomyelinase-deficient macrophages: implications for Niemann-Pick disease enzyme replacement therapy. J Biol Chem 279(2): 1526-32

Dodge JC, Clarke J, Song A, Bu J, Yang W, Taksir TV, Griffiths D, Zhao MA, Schuchman EH, Cheng SH, O' Riordan CR, Shihabuddin LS, Passini MA, Stewart GR. 2005. Gene transfer of human acid sphingomyelinase corrects neuropathology and motor deficits in a mouse model of Niemann-Pick type A disease. Proc Natl Acad Sci U S A 102(49): 17822-7

Frolov A, Zielinski SE, Crowley JR, Dudley-Rucker N, Schaffer JE, Ory DS. 2003. NPC1 and NPC2 regulate cellular cholesterol homeostasis through generation of low density lipoprotein cholesterol-derived oxysterols. J Biol Chem 278(28): 25517-25

Gelsthorpe ME, Baumann N, Millard E, Gale SE, Langmade SJ, Schaffer JE, Ory DS. 2008. Niemann-Pick type C1 I1061T mutant encodes a functional protein that is selected for endoplasmic reticulum-associated degradation due to protein misfolding. J Biol Chem 283(13): 8229-36

Göritz C, Mauch DH, Nägler K, Pfrieger FW. 2002. Role of glia-derived cholesterol in synaptogenesis: new revelations in the synapse-glia affair. J Physiol Paris 96(3-4): 257-63

Gondré-Lewis MC, McGlynn R, Walkley SU. 2003. Cholesterol accumulation in NPC1-deficient neurons is ganglioside dependent. Curr Biol 13(15): 1324-9

Horinouchi K, Erlich S, Perl DP, Ferlinz K, Bisgaier CL, Sandhoff K, Desnick RJ, Stewart CL, Schuchman EH. 1995. Acid sphingomyelinase deficient mice: a model of types A and B Niemann-Pick disease. Nat Genet 10(3): 288-93

Lachmann RH, te Vruchte D, Lloyd-Evans E, Reinkensmeier G, Sillence DJ, Fernandez-Guillen L, Dwek RA, Butters TD, Cox TM, Platt FM. 2004. Treatment with miglustat reverses the lipid-trafficking defect in Niemann-Pick disease type C. Neurobiol Dis 16(3): 654-8

Liu B, Turley SD, Burns DK, Miller AM, Repa JJ, Dietschy JM. 2009. Reversal of defective lysosomal transport in NPC disease ameliorates liver dysfunction and neurodegeneration in the npc1-/-mouse. Proc Natl Acad Sci U S A 106(7): 2377-82

Lloyd-Evans E, Morgan AJ, He X, Smith DA, Elliot-Smith E, Sillence DJ, Churchill GC, Schuchman EH, Galione A, Platt FM. 2008. Niemann-Pick disease type C1 is a sphingosine storage disease that causes deregulation of lysosomal calcium. Nat Med 14(11): 1247-55

Loftus SK, Morris JA, Carstea ED, Gu JZ, Cummings C, Brown A, Ellison J, Ohno K, Rosenfeld MA, Tagle DA, Pentchev PG, Pavan WJ. 1997. Murine model of Niemann-Pick C disease: mutation in a cholesterol homeostasis gene. Science 277(5323): 232-5

Millat G, Marçais C, Tomasetto C, Chikh K, Fensom AH, Harzer K, Wenger DA, Ohno K, Vanier MT. 2001. Niemann-Pick C1 disease: correlations between NPC1 mutations, levels of NPC1 protein, and phenotypes emphasize the functional significance of the putative sterol-sensing domain and of the cysteine-rich luminal loop. Am J Hum Genet 68(6): 1373-85

Miranda SR, He X, Simonaro CM, Gatt S, Dagan A, Desnick RJ, Schuchman EH. 2000. Infusion of recombinant human acid sphingomyelinase into niemann-pick disease mice leads to visceral, but not neurological, correction of the pathophysiology. FASEB J 14(13): 1988-95

Naureckiene S, Sleat DE, Lackland H, Fensom A, Vanier MT, Wattiaux R, Jadot M, Lobel P. 2000. Identification of HE1 as the second gene of Niemann-Pick C disease. Science 290(5500): 2298-301

Passini MA, Macauley SL, Huff MR, Taksir TV, Bu J, Wu IH, Piepenhagen PA, Dodge JC, Shihabuddin LS, O' Riordan CR, Schuchman EH, Stewart GR. 2005. AAV vector-mediated correction of brain pathology in a mouse model of Niemann-Pick A disease. Mol Ther 11(5): 754-62

Patterson MC, Vecchio D, Prady H, Abel L, Wraith JE. 2007. Miglustat for treatment of Niemann-Pick C disease: a randomised controlled study. Lancet Neurol 6(9): 765-72

Repa JJ, Li H, Frank-Cannon TC, Valasek MA, Turley SD, Tansey MG, Dietschy JM. 2007. Liver X receptor activation enhances cholesterol loss from the brain, decreases neuroinflammation, and increases survival of the NPC1 mouse. J Neurosci 27(52): 14470-80

Quintern LE, Schuchman EH, Levran O, Suchi M, Ferlinz K, Reinke H, Sandhoff K, Desnick RJ. 1989. Isolation of cDNA clones encoding human acid sphingomyelinase: occurrence of alternatively processed transcripts. EMBO J 8(9): 2469-73

Ries M, Schaefer E, Lührs T, Mani L, Kuhn J, Vanier MT, Krummenauer F, Gal A, Beck M, Mengel E. 2006. Critical assessment of chitotriosidase analysis in the rational laboratory diagnosis of children with Gaucher disease and Niemann-Pick disease type A/B and C. J Inherit Metab Dis 29(5): 647-52

Schuchman EH, Levran O, Pereira LV, Desnick RJ. 1992. Structural organization and complete nucleotide sequence of the gene encoding human acid sphingomyelinase (SMPD1). Genomics 12(2): 197-205

Sleat DE, Wiseman JA, El-Banna M, Price SM, Verot L, Shen MM, Tint GS, Vanier MT, Walkley SU, Lobel P. 2004. Genetic evidence for nonredundant functional cooperativity between NPC1 and NPC2 in lipid transport. Proc Natl Acad Sci U S A 101(16): 5886-91

Smith EL, Schuchman EH. 2008. The unexpected role of acid sphingomyelinase in cell death and the pathophysiology of common diseases. FASEB J 22(10): 3419-31

Sturley SL, Patterson MC, Pentchev P. 2009. Unraveling the sterol-trafficking defect in Niemann-Pick C disease. Proc Natl Acad Sci U S A 106(7): 2093-4

Trinh MN, Brown MS, Seemann J, Goldstein JL, Lu F. 2018. Lysosomal cholesterol export reconstituted from fragments of Niemann-Pick C1. Elife 7: e38564

Van Diggelen OP, Voznyi YV, Keulemans JL, Schoonderwoerd K, Ledvinova J, Mengel E, Zschiesche M, Santer R, Harzer K. 200. A new fluorimetric enzyme assay for the diagnosis of Niemann-Pick A/B, with specificity of natural sphingomyelinase substrate. J Inherit Metab Dis 28(5): 733-41

Vanier MT, Rodriguez-Lafrasse C, Rousson R, Mandon G, Boué J, Choiset A, Peyrat MF, Dumontel C, Juge MC, Pentchev PG, et al. 1992. Prenatal diagnosis of Niemann-Pick type C disease: current strategy from an experience of 37 pregnancies at risk. Am J Hum Genet 51(1): 111-22

Vanier MT, Duthel S, Rodriguez-Lafrasse C, Pentchev P, Carstea ED. 1996. Genetic heterogeneity in Niemann-Pick C disease: a study using somatic cell hybridization and linkage analysis. Am J Hum Genet 58(1): 118-25

Vanier MT. 1999. Lipid changes in Niemann-Pick disease type C brain: personal experience and review of the literature. Neurochem Res 24(4): 481-9

Wasserstein, M., R. Lachmann, C. Hollak, L. Arash-Kaps, A. Barbato, R. C. Gallagher, R. Giugliani, N. B. Guelbert, T. Ikezoe, O. Lidove, P. Mabe, E. Mengel, M. Scarpa, E. Senates, M. Tchan, J. Villarrubia, Y. Chen, S. Furey, B. L. Thurberg, A. Zaher and M. Kumar 2022. A randomized, placebo-controlled clinical trial evaluating olipudase alfa enzyme replacement therapy for chronic acid sphingomyelinase deficiency (ASMD) in adults: One-year results. Genet Med. 24: 1425-1436

Winkler MBL, Kidmose RT, Szomek M, Thaysen K, Rawson S, Muench SP, Wüstner D, Pedersen BP. 2019. Structural Insight into Eukaryotic Sterol Transport through Niemann-Pick Type C Proteins. Cell 179(2): 485-497.e1

Zervas M, Dobrenis K, Walkley SU. 2001. Neurons in Niemann-Pick disease type C accumulate gangliosides as well as unesterified cholesterol and undergo dendritic and axonal alterations. J Neuropathol Exp Neurol 60(1): 49-64

Genetics of Niemann-Pick disease

3. Genetics of Niemann-Pick disease

In 1961, Crocker et al. (1961) defined four clinical subgroups of Niemann-Pick disease:

- Type A: an acute neuronopathic form (classic infantile)
- Type B: a chronic form without neurological involvement (visceral)
- Type C: a chronic neuronopathic form
- Type D: the so-called "Nova Scotia variant"

Two further forms appeared in the course of the 1970s: type E, an adult, non-neuronopathic form and type F, a heat-dependent variant of type A/B. As shown in the other chapters of this textbook, such a classification system can hardly be justified today due to the extraordinary variability in Niemann-Pick disease and the many overlaps between the subgroups. Rather than expanding the clinical classification system, the forms of the Niemann-Pick disease – thanks in particular to considerable advances in genetics – were classified into two metabolic diseases with so far three disease-associated genes:

- Niemann-Pick disease types A/B (NPA/B), caused by reduced acid sphingomyelinase (ASM) activity due to defects in the *SMPD1* gene, and
- Niemann-Pick disease type C (NPC), caused by impairment of the lipid transport protein due to defects in the *NPC1* or *NPC2* gene.

3.1. Niemann-Pick disease type A/B (NPA/B) [MIM: 257200/607616]

A familial cause for Niemann-Pick disease was assumed as early as 1916 when two siblings were diagnosed with the disease (Knox et al 1916). Autosomal recessive inheritance was suggested at an early stage based on the equal distribution among boys and girls as well as the increased occurrence among children of blood relatives (Siegmund 1921; Crocker et al. 1958). Niemann-Pick disease types A and B have been described in all ethnic groups. The incidence observed in different populations fluctuates between 0.3 and 0.6 per 100,000 births (Giugliani et al. 2017). Type A occurs very frequently in Ashkenazi Jews. The carrier frequency in the Jewish population is given as 1:80, which means that the incidence of the disease is around 1:40,000 (Goodman 1979). Both NPA and NPB are rare in the non-Jewish population, and NPB has a significantly higher prevalence than NPA. This is especially true for people of Turkish, Arab and North African origin (Vanier et al. 1993; Simonaro et al. 2002).

3.1.1. *SMPD1* gene and ASM protein [HGNC Gene-ID: 11120]

As early as 1966, Brady et al. decoded the metabolic defect of NPA disease as a deficiency in acid sphingomyelinase (ASM) enzyme activity (Brady et al. 1966), shortly after it was purified and characterized from rat liver (Kanfer et al. 1966). The first cDNA constructs of this enzyme were not described until 20 years later (Quintern et al. 1989). Several alternative splice products included a transcript with a length of 1.890 base pairs (bp) which encoded a protein with enzymatic activity (Schuchman et al. 1991).

The ASM protein (UniProt ID: P17405) consists of 631 amino acids and is composed of a saposin binding region, a proline-rich region, a metal phosphatase and a C-terminal domain. It contains six potential glycosylation sites, eight disulfide bridges and two zinc ions, which play a crucial role in the folding and stabilization of the protein (Zhou et al. 2016). After synthesis in the endoplasmic reticulum and subsequent glycosylation, the 72 kDa mature protein is transported into lysosomes; a small amount of ASM is secreted.

The ASM protein is encoded by the *SMPD1* gene, which codes for 6 exons with a length of 77 to 773 bp and extends over 5 kilobases (kb) on chromosome 11p15.1-p15.4. About 44% of the ASM protein is encoded by exon 2. The GC-rich promoter region contains potential binding sites for the transcription factors SP1, TAT, CAAT, NF-1 and AP-1 (Schuchman et al. 1992).

3.1.2. *SMPD1* variants

The clinical manifestation of NPA/B disease correlates directly with the degree of inhibition of acid sphingomyelinase (ASM). If the enzyme activity falls below approximately 5% residual activity, a severe course of the NPA disease can be assumed. If, on the other hand, the enzyme activity is only reduced to less than 10% residual activity, NPB symptoms are to be expected. ASM enzyme activity is in turn largely determined by the genetic defect present in each case (Schuchman and Desnick 2001). Frameshift mutations, larger or small insertions and deletions as well as faulty splicing usually reduce enzyme activity the most and are typically associated with NPA. The simultaneous presence of two type A mutations therefore generally allows the prediction of a severe neurodegenerative disease pattern with onset at an early age.

The designation of the gene variants mentioned here follows the current HGVS guidelines (Human Genome Variation Society; den Dunnen et al. 2016). It should be noted that the nomenclature of the *SMD1* mutations was previously based on a different cDNA sequence: Since the reference sequence in exon 1 contains a highly polymorphic hexanucleotide sequence that is repeated three to eight times, *SMD1* mutations located from nucleotide 142 (amino acid 48) downwards can be described in two different ways, which are listed in Table S1 of the publication by Zampierei et al. (Zampieri et al. 2016).

More than 90% of all NPA variants present in the Ashkenazi Jewish population can be traced back to only three *SMPD1* alleles. Firstly, there is the frame-shift mutation p.F333Sfx52 (Levran et al. 1993), which leads to a premature stop codon and is, if homozygous, usually fatal in early childhood. The other two common variants are the missense mutations p.L304P and p.R498L (Levran et al. 1991a; Levran et al. 1992), the base exchange leading to p.R498L taking place in a CpG dinucleotide that represents a known mutation hotspot. "Non-Jewish" Type A mutations are usually private mutations and distributed throughout the coding region of the *SMPD1* gene. Their relative accumulation in exon 3 is attributed to its role in coding the catalytic center of the ASM enzyme.

A common NPB mutation with high residual enzymatic activity is p.R610del, which leads to the deletion of three base pairs and is particularly common in patients in North Africa (Vanier et al. 1993). A patient with compound heterozygosity for p.R610del together with the "type A mutation" p.R498L showed only a mild course of the disease similar to NPB (Levran et al. 1991b). Common alleles in Turkish NPB patients are p.L139P, p.S192fs*1 and p.L551P, and the change p.H423Y associated with severe NPB disease was found in around 70% of all patients from Saudi Arabia (Simonaro et al. 2002). The mutations p.R3AfsX76 and p.H284SfsX7 were predominantly detected in Chinese NPA/B patients (Zhang et al. 2013).

For most of the mutations described, there is a significant, but not complete correlation between genotype and phenotype (Desnick et al. 2010). It should be noted here that the *SMPD1* gene can be subject to paternal imprinting, which means that the maternally inherited maternal allele is predominantly expressed. As a result, the clinical characteristics of a patient mainly correlate with the sphingomyelinase activity that is expressed by the maternal mutation (Simonaro et al. 2006; Ceron-Rodriguez et al. 2019).

In addition to disease-associated mutations, the coding region of the *SMPD1* gene contains several non-synonymous polymorphisms with unknown disease relevance, e.g. p.V36A, p.V318E, p.T323I and p.G508R. In addition, the number of alanine and leucine repeats in the region coding for the signal peptide can vary (Schuchman and Desnick 2001).

3.2. Niemann-Pick disease type C (NPC) [MIM: 257220/607625]

In contrast to patients with NPA and NPB, tissue and cultured fibroblasts from patients who were assigned to the clinical forms type C and type D showed an inconspicuous or only slightly reduced enzyme activity of acid sphingomyelinase (Schneider and Kennedy 1967), which was increasingly interpreted as being a secondary effect. Since the reduced enzyme activity of type A/B cells could be complemented by fusion with cells from type C/D patients, Besley et al. postulated the existence of at least one other Niemann-Pick gene in 1980 (Besley et al. 1980).

In order to calculate the incidence of Niemann-Pick disease type C, Wassif et al. collected data on the allele frequency in different ethnic groups from four large databases. 17,754 chromosomes could be analyzed for the presence of a (heterozygous) mutation in the NPC1 or NPC2 gene (Wassif et al. 2016). From the number of detected pathogenic variants, an incidence of 1:92.104 for Niemann-

Pick disease type C1 and 1:2,858,998 for Niemann-Pick disease type C2 was calculated using the Hardy-Weinberg formula. The combined incidence of NPC1 and NPC2 is 1:89.229 or 1.12 cases per 100,000 births. The late-onset NPC1 phenotype is probably much more common at 1:19,000 to 1:36,000 (Wassif et al. 2016). The incidence rates found in different countries vary between 0.25 and 2.20 per 100,000 births (Geberhiwot 2018). In some populations, for example in Nova Scotia, New Mexico and on a small Greek island, the incidence of NPC1 is much higher due to a founder effect (Seker Yilmaz et al. 2020).

The vast majority (~95%) of patients with Niemann-Pick type C (NPC) have mutations in the *NPC1* gene. The main characteristics of the three genes associated with Niemann-Pick diseases are shown in Table 3.1.

3.2.1. *NPC1* gene and protein [HGNC Gene-ID: 7897]

In the early 1990s, more than 30 families with clinical type C, in which Pentchev et al. had found an impaired formation of cholesterol esters after stimulation with LDL (Pentchev et al. 1987), participated in a large-scale linkage study. As a result, the disease-associated NPC locus could be narrowed down to the pericentric region of chromosome 18 (Carstea et al. 1993). With the help of complementation experiments in which fragments of human chromosome 18 were introduced into 3T3 cells of NPC mice, the cellular disease phenotype (the massive storage of free cholesterol in lysosomes) could be corrected by fragments of the region 18q11-q12. Linkage analyses of members of the Niemann-Pick families in Nova Scotia showed that the previously assumed NPD locus overlapped with the NPC locus, which can only mean that these must be different manifestations

HGNC gene symbol	SMPD1	NPC1	NPC2
Associated clinical picture	NP-A MIM: 257200 NP-B MIM: 607616	NPC1 MIM: 257220	NPC2 MIM: 607625
Aliases	ASM	—	HE-1, EDDM1
HGNC gene name	sphingomyelin phosphodiesterase 1, acid lysosomal	Niemann-Pick disease, type C1	Niemann-Pick disease, type C2
Enzyme nomenclature	3.1.4.41	no enzyme	no enzyme
HGNC gene ID	11120	7897	14537
Chromosomal localization	11p15.4-p15.1	18q11-q12	14q24.3
NCBI Entrez Gene ID	6609	4864	10577
Genomic localization	chr11:6,411,655-6,416,225	chr18:21,111,464-21,166,581	chr14:74,946,644-74,960,084
Gene size	4,571 bp	55,118 bp	13,441 bp
Number of exons	6	25	5
Number of RefSeq isoforms	3	1	1
Reference transcript ID	NM_000543	NM_000271	NM_006432
Reference transcript mRNA size	2,458 bp	4,812 bp	896 bp
Gene product	acid sphingomyelin phosphodiesterase 1	Niemann-Pick type C1 protein (NPC1)	Niemann-Pick type C2 protein (NPC2)
UniProt ID	P17405	O15118	P61916
Reference protein size	631 aa	1278 aa	151 aa
Subcellular localization	lysosomes, secretory	late endosomes, lysosomes, TGN	late endosomes, lysosomes, secretory

Table 3.1: Niemann-Pick genes by comparison.

of the same clinical picture (Greer et al. 1997). Linkage analyses in a consanguineous Arab family allowed a further narrowing down of the interval between the markers D18S44 and D18S1388, a 1-cM region that could be imaged by three artificial yeast chromosomes, one of which complemented the disease phenotype. Sequencing of the corresponding region in patients revealed mutations in a gene which had also been deleted in the NPC^{nih} mouse model and whose 4.673 bp long cDNA complemented the disease phenotype in patient cells (Carstea et al. 1997).

This *NPC1* gene extends to 56 kb on chromosome 18q11-q12 and codes for 25 exons with sizes between 74 and 788 bp. NPC1 orthologues show a high degree of homology: 85% of the amino acids in the mouse, 34% in yeast and 30% in *Caenorhabditis elegans* are identical to the human NPC1 protein. The 5'-untranslated region and intron 1 contain CpG islands with several potential binding sites for the transcription factor Sp1. *NPC1* is expressed in all tissues and codes for a membrane protein of 1,278 amino acids (aa) with a molecular weight of 142 kDa. At the N-terminus there is a targeting signal for protein synthesis in the endoplasmic reticulum, while the cytoplasmic C-terminus carries a dileucin motif (LLNF), which ensures the transport into late endosomes and lysosomes. Amino acids 73-94 correspond to a leucine zipper motif. The NPC1 protein has 14 potential glycosylation sites and a tyrosine residue at position 506 can be phosphorylated. The post-translational modifications lead to a molecular weight of around 170-190 kDa (Patterson et al. 2001; Vanier and Millat 2003). Five of the total of 13 transmembrane domains (TMD 3-7; aa 615-797) represent a so-called sterol-sensing domain, as is also found in other proteins with important functions in cellular cholesterol regulation (e.g. in HMG-CoA reductase, SCAP and NPC1L1) and the protein Patched (Davies and Ioannou 2000). Three large luminal loop domains are obviously of functional relevance: The N-terminal Loop1 domain (aa 25-264) is highly conserved and has sterol binding properties. The domain itself does not seem to be essential for the cholesterol-transporting function of NPC1; however, due to a disproportionately higher affinity for 25-hydroxycholesterol relative to cholesterol, an important regulatory function is assumed (Infante et al. 2008; Kwon et al. 2009). The pathogenetically relevant Loop3 domain between TMD 8 and 9 (aa 855-1098), the so-called cysteine-rich domain (Greer et al. 1999), has a sequence homology to the RING finger motif of protein kinase C and contains approximately 30% of the disease-causing NPC1 mutation (☞ below).

In cells, native NPC1 protein is found on the membranes of intraluminal vesicles and, in particular, on the limiting membrane of late endosomes and lysosomes. NPC1 can also be detected in smaller amounts in the trans-Golgi apparatus and in endoplasmic reticulum-associated transport vesicles (Karten et al. 2009).

3.2.2. *NPC1* variants

So far, around 500 sequence variants have been detected in the *NPC1* gene (Dardis et al. 2020). The variants are distributed over the entire range of the coding sequence of *NPC1* and are private in the majority of cases. Most NPC patients in Western countries therefore show compound heterozygosity for previously not at all or only rarely described variants, which makes predictions both about the disease relevance of newly identified sequence variants and the expected course of the disease considerably more difficult. Most of the variants described are missense mutations. A large percentage of these can be detected in the cysteine-rich Loop3 domain. p.I1061T is the most common *NPC1* mutation and is found in around 20% of all Western European NPC patients (Vanier and Millat 2003; Runz et al. 2008). The mutation p.G992W was identified as the cause of the Nova Scotia variant of Niemann-Pick disease classified as type D (Greer et al. 1998). The cases observed so far suggest a certain genotype/phenotype correlation: Mutations within the sterol-sensitive domain of the NPC1 protein seem to cause the most severe functional impairment, as they generally correlate with a rapidly progressive infantile course of disease (Millat et al. 2001b). Variants in this domain do not only significantly restrict the further distribution of LDL cholesterol to the plasma membrane and the ER, but also significantly reduce the binding affinity of a photo-activatable cholesterol analog (Millard et al. 2005). The variant p.R518W was detected in several adult patients and was therefore associated with a rather mild course of the disease (Ribeiro et al. 2001; Runz et al. 2008).

However, genotype-phenotype correlations are not always reliable. Homozygosity for the mutation p.I1061T was originally described as being associated with a late infantile course of the disease (Millat et al. 1999), but could later also be found in patients with an early infantile clinical picture. In addition, heterozygosity for p.I1061T is found in patients with all forms of the disease (Battisti et al. 2003; Imrie et al. 2007). The presence of a very severe mutation (frameshift, nonsense, large deletion) on both alleles leads to an early infantile neurological disease or to an – often fatal – systemic manifestation in newborns. Some missense mutations in homozygous form, such as the mutation p.G1240R, can also be responsible for a severe course. The missense mutations p.R978C, p.G992R and p.D874V are mainly associated with a late-onset neurological course of the Niemann-Pick C1 disease, even if there is a nonsense mutation on the second allele (Geberhiwot et al. 2018). The mutation p.P1007A is also frequently observed in juvenile or adult patients, and less often in late-infantile patients. If this gene change is present on both or even only one allele, the filipin test can be very weak, which makes the interpretation of this test for diagnosis more difficult (Millat et al. 2001b). The mutation p.H215R appears to be a risk factor for the development of obesity (den Hoed et al. 2013).

Synonymous and non-synonymous single nucleotide polymorphisms (SNPs) are found with high frequency in the *NPC1* gene: The most common polymorphisms in families of Central European origin are p.Y129Y (rs12970899), p.H215R (rs1805081), p.M642I (rs1788799), p.I858V (rs1805082) and p.N931N (rs7229671; Bauer et al. 2002; Vanier and Millat 2003; Runz et al. 2008). With a population frequency of up to 5%, p.P237S appears to be a polymorphism that is particularly common in the Scandinavian population, and the variant p.R1266Q (rs1805084) is also found in healthy controls.

3.2.3. *NPC2* gene and protein [HGNC Gene-ID: 14537]

Naureckiene and co-workers discovered mutations in the *HE1* gene in NPC2 patients, which codes for the secretory protein HE1 detectable in the human epididymis, and were thus able to demonstrate that the *NPC2* gene for the Niemann-Pick type 2 disease is identical to the *HE1* gene (Naureckiene et al. 2000). The *NPC2* (or *HE1*) gene is located on the long arm of chromosome 14 (14q24.3). It is 13.5 kb long and composed of 5 exons. It is expressed in all tissues and codes for a small secretory protein 151 amino acids in length. After cleavage of a 19 amino acid long signal peptide in the endoplasmic reticulum, the protein is heavily glycosylated and can be released into the extracellular space via the secretory route (Xu et al. 2019). However, glycosylated NPC2 also binds to the mannose-6-phosphate receptor, which enables transport into lysosomal compartments, with smaller amounts also being present in endosomal compartments and in the Golgi apparatus (Storch and Xu 2009). In a hydrophobic binding domain, the NPC2 protein directly binds cholesterol and numerous other lipids (Xu et al. 2019) and has other domains of potentially functional relevance. It is generally accepted that the function of NPC1 and NPC2 is not redundant, but that both proteins play a concerted role in the export of cholesterol and other lipids from late endosomes and lysosomes (Storch and Xu 2009; Kwon et al. 2009).

3.2.4. *NPC2* variants

There are currently 28 known mutations of the *NPC2* gene. Of these, 19 are missense/nonsense mutations, four are splice site variants, three are small deletions, one is an insertion/deletion and one is a large deletion (Seker Yilmaz et al. 2020). There is a certain genotype/phenotype correlation. Large deletions, frame shifts, stop codon mutations and mutations of the initiation codon lead to a severe, early fatal course of the disease. These are, for example, the mutations p.M1L, p.M1I, p.L9fs, p.E20X, p.E118X and others. The IVS2 + 5G> A, V39M, and P120S mutations are observed in adolescent or adult patients with neurological manifestations (Millat et al. 2001a; Xu et al. 2019).

3.3. Challenges of genetic testing in Niemann-Pick disease and outlook

If the presence of two known mutations can be demonstrated in a patient with suspected Niemann-Pick molecular genetics, the diagnostic reliability is very high, so that the expected course of the disease can be reliably predicted for some mutation combinations. To confirm the diagnosis of NPA/B, especially in the non-Jewish population, the determination of ASM enzyme activity from isolated leukocytes and/or fibroblast cultures is preferable to genetic diagnosis, since the remaining activity generally correlates well with the clinical picture. In the case of heterozygosity, however, biochemical testing is unreliable, so that a molecular genetic test is preferable to check for carrier status. The three relevant *SMPD1* mutations at Ashkenazim are specifically examined in population screening, and direct-to-consumer tests are also available (e.g. at Counsyl [http://www.counsyl.com]). For prenatal examinations, genetic *SMPD1* diagnostics are often associated with advantages if the mutation status of the parents is known. NPB patients with homozygosity or compound heterozygosity for the *SMPD1* mutation p.Q292K show normal or even slightly increased ASM enzyme activity when using an artificial sphingomyelinase substrate that is often used in routine diagnostics, which carries the risk of false-negative results (Harzer et al. 2003).

In accordance with current recommendations, a molecular genetic test must be carried out in addition to the filipin test, including an examination of the parents for segregation analysis, if Niemann-Pick disease type C is suspected (Geberhiwot et al. 2018). However, in about 12-15% of the cases, it is not possible to detect mutations in both alleles of the *NPC1* or *NPC2* gene using standard methods (Wassif et al. 2016). For example, the identification of mutations of the intron or promoter or of large deletions/duplications may require further genetic testing, such as the analysis of the gDNA and cDNA or the application of the MLPA (multiplex ligation-dependent probe amplification; Vanier et al. 2016). In any case, all molecular biological methods should be exhausted in patients in whom the symptoms strongly suspect the presence of Niemann-Pick disease type C, even if the filipin test (as is often the case with the mutation p.P1007A) shows no clear result (Patterson et al. 2012).

However, if a mutation can only be detected on one allele in a patient with only mild neurological symptoms, there is also the possibility that he is actually heterozygous. In recent years, patients with symptoms of a neurodegenerative disease such as Parkinson's disease, Alzheimer's disease or corticobasal degeneration have been observed (Klünemann et al. 2013; Cupidi et al. 2017). In some of them, morphological and metabolic changes in the central nervous system could be determined by means of MRI and SPECT examinations (Cupidi et al. 2017).

3.4. Genetic databases for Niemann-Pick diseases

- HGMD:
  http://www.hgmd.org
- UniProt:
  http://www.uniprot.org

References

Battisti C, Tarugi P, Dotti MT, De Stefano N, Vattimo A, Chierichetti F, Calandra S, Federico A. 2003. Adult onset Niemann-Pick type C disease: A clinical, neuroimaging and molecular genetic study. Mov Disord 18: 1405

Bauer P, Knoblich R, Bauer C, Finckh U, Hufen A, Kropp J, Braun S, Kustermann-Kuhn B, Schmidt D, Harzer K, Rolfs A. 2002. NPC1: Complete genomic sequence, mutation analysis, and characterization of haplotypes. Hum Mutat 19: 30

Besley GT, Hoogeboom AJ, Hoogeveen A, Kleijer WJ, Galjaard H. 1980. Somatic cell hybridization studies showing different gene mutations in Niemann-Pick variants. Hum Genet 54: 409

Brady RO, Kanfer JN, Mock MB, Fredrickson DS. 1966.The metabolism of sphingomyelin II. Evidence of an enzymatic deficiency in Niemann-Pick disease. Proc Natl Acad Sci USA 55: 366

Carstea ED, Morris JA, Coleman KG, Loftus SK, Zhang D, Cummings C, Gu J, Rosenfeld MA, Pavan WJ, Krizman DB, Nagle J, Polymeropoulos MH, Sturley SL, Ioannou YA, Higgins ME, Comly M, Cooney A, Brown A, Kaneski CR, Blanchette-Mackie EJ, Dwyer NK, Neufeld EB, Chang TY, Liscum L, Strauss JF 3rd, Ohno K, Zeigler M, Carmi R, Sokol J, Markie D, O'Neill RR, van Diggelen OP, Elleder M, Patterson MC, Brady RO, Vanier MT, Pentchev PG, Tagle DA. 1997. Niemann-Pick C1 disease gene: homology to mediators of cholesterol homeostasis. Science 277: 228

Carstea ED, Polymeropoulos MH, Parker CC, Detera-Wadleigh SD, O'Neill RR, Patterson MC, Goldin E, Xiao H, Straub RE, Vanier MT, et al. 1993. Linkage of Niemann-Pick disease type C to human chromosome 18. Proc Natl Acad Sci USA 90: 2002

Ceron-Rodriguez M, Vazquez-Martinez ER, Garcia-Delgado C, Ortega-Vazquez A, Valencia-Mayoral P, Ramirez-Devars L, Arias-Villegas C, Monroy-Munoz IE, Lopez M, Cervantes A, Cerbon M, Moran-Barroso VF.

2019. Niemann-Pick disease A or B in four pediatric patients and SMPD1 mutation carrier frequency in the Mexican population. Ann Hepatol 18: 613

Crocker A, Farber S. 1958. Niemann-Pick disease: A review of eighteen patients. Medicine (Baltimore) 37: 1

Crocker A. 1961. The cerebral defect in Tay Sachs disease and Niemann-Pick disease. J Neurochem 7: 69

Cupidi C, Frangipane F, Gallo M, Clodomiro A, Colao R, Bernardi L, Anfossi M, Conidi ME, Vasso F, Curcio SA, Mirabelli M, Smirne N, Torchia G, Muraca MG, Puccio G, Di Lorenzo R, Zampieri S, Romanello M, Dardis A, Maletta RG, Bruni AC. 2017. Role of Niemann-Pick Type C Disease Mutations in Dementia. J Alzheimers Dis 55: 1249

Dardis A, Zampieri S, Gellera C, Carrozzo R, Cattarossi S, Peruzzo P, Dariol R, Sechi A, Deodato F, Caccia C, Verrigni D, Gasperini S, Fiumara A, Fecarotta S, Carecchio M, Filosto M, Santoro L, Borroni B, Bordugo A, Brancati F, Russo CV, Di Rocco M, Toscano A, Scarpa M, Bembi B. 2020. Molecular Genetics of Niemann-Pick Type C Disease in Italy: An Update on 105 Patients and Description of 18 NPC1 Novel Variants. J Clin Med 9: 679

Davies JP, Ioannou YA. 2000. Topological analysis of Niemann-Pick C1 protein reveals that the membrane orientation of the putative sterol-sensing domain is identical to those of 3-hydroxy-3-methylglutaryl-CoA reductase and sterol regulatory element binding protein cleavage-activating protein. J Biol Chem 275: 24367

den Dunnen JT, Dalgleish R, Maglott DR, Hart RK, Greenblatt MS, McGowan-Jordan J, Roux A-F, Smith T, Antonarakis SE, Taschner PEM. 2016. HGVS Recommendations for the Description of Sequence Variants: 2016 Update. Human Mutation 37: 564

den Hoed M, Luan J, Langenberg C, Cooper C, Sayer AA, Jameson K, Kumari M, Kivimaki M, Hingorani AD, Grontved A, Khaw KT, Ekelund U, Wareham NJ, Loos RJ. 2013. Evaluation of common genetic variants identified by GWAS for early onset and morbid obesity in population-based samples. Int J Obes (Lond) 37: 191

Desnick JP, Kim J, He X, Wasserstein MP, Simonaro CM, Schuchman EH. 2010. Identification and characterization of eight novel SMPD1 mutations causing types A and B Niemann-Pick disease. Mol Med 16: 316

Geberhiwot T, Moro A, Dardis A, Ramaswami U, Sirrs S, Marfa MP, Vanier MT, Walterfang M, Bolton S, Dawson C, Heron B, Stampfer M, Imrie J, Hendriksz C, Gissen P, Crushell E, Coll MJ, Nadjar Y, Klunemann H, Mengel E, Hrebicek M, Jones SA, Ory D, Bembi B, Patterson M, International Niemann-Pick Disease R. 2018. Consensus clinical management guidelines for Niemann-Pick disease type C. Orphanet J Rare Dis 13: 50

Giugliani R, Federhen A, Michelin-Tirelli K, Riegel M, Burin M. 2017. Relative frequency and estimated minimal frequency of Lysosomal Storage Diseases in Brazil: Report from a Reference Laboratory. Genet Mol Biol 40: 31

Goodman R. 1979. Genetic disorders among the Jewish people. Baltimore, Johns Hopkins University Press

Greer WL, Riddell DC, Byers DM, Welch JP, Girouard GS, Sparrow SM, Gillan TL, Neumann PE. 1997. Linkage of Niemann-Pick disease type D to the same region of human chromosome 18 as Niemann-Pick disease type C. Am J Hum Genet. 61: 139

Greer WL, Dobson MJ, Girouard GS, Byers DM, Riddell DC, Neumann PE. 1999. Mutations in NPC1 highlight a conserved NPC1-specific cysteine-rich domain. Am J Hum Genet 65: 1252

Greer WL, Riddell DC, Gillan TL, Girouard GS, Sparrow SM, Byers DM, Dobson MJ, Neumann PE. 1998. The Nova Scotia (type D) form of Niemann-Pick disease is caused by a G3097->T transversion in NPC1. Am J Hum Genet 63: 52

Harzer K, Rolfs A, Bauer P, Zschiesche M, Mengel E, Backes J, Kustermann-Kuhn B, Bruchelt G, van Diggelen OP, Mayrhofer H, Krägeloh-Mann I. 2003. Niemann-Pick disease type A and B are clinically but also enzymatically heterogeneous: pitfall in the laboratory diagnosis of sphingomyelinase deficiency associated with the mutation Q292 K. Neuropediatrics 34: 301

Imrie J, Dasgupta S, Besley GT, Harris C, Heptinstall L, Knight S, Vanier MT, Fensom AH, Ward C, Jacklin E, Whitehouse C, Wraith JE. 2007. The natural history of Niemann-Pick disease type C in the UK. J Inherit Metab Dis 30: 51

Infante RE, Radhakrishnan A, Abi-Mosleh L, Kinch LN, Wang ML, Grishin NV, Goldstein JL, Brown MS. 2008. Purified NPC1 protein: II. Localization of sterol binding to a 240-amino acid soluble luminal loop. J Biol Chem 283: 1064

Kanfer JN, Young OM, Shapiro D, Brady RO. 1966. The metabolism of sphingomyelin I. Purification and properties of a sphingomyelin-cleaving enzyme from rat liver tissue. J Biol Chem 241: 1081

Karten B, Peake KB, Vance JE. 2009. Mechanisms and consequences of impaired lipid trafficking in Niemann-Pick type C1-deficient mammalian cells. Biochim Biophys Acta 1791: 659

Klünemann HH, Nutt JG, Davis MY, Bird TD. 2013. Parkinsonism syndrome in heterozygotes for Niemann-Pick C1. J Neurol Sci 335: 219

Knox J, Wahl W, Schmeisser A. 1916. Gaucher's disease in infants. Bull Johns Hopkins Hosp 27: 1

Kwon HJ, Abi-Mosleh L, Wang ML, Deisenhofer J, Goldstein JL, Brown MS, Infante RE. 2009. Structure of N-terminal domain of NPC1 reveals distinct subdomains for binding and transfer of cholesterol. Cell 137: 1213

Levran O, Desnick RJ, Schuchman EH. 1991a. Niemann-Pick disease: A frequent missense mutation in the acid spingomyelinase gene of Ashkenazi Jewish type A and B patients. Proc Natl Acad Sci USA 88: 3748

Levran O, Desnick RJ, Schuchman EH. 1992. A common missense mutation (L302P) in Ashkenazi Jewish type A Niemann-Pick disease patients. Blood 80: 2081

Levran O, Desnick RJ, Schuchman EH. 1993. Type A Niemann-Pick disease: A frameshift mutation in the acid sphingomyelinase gene (fsP330) occurs in Ashkenazi Jewish patients, Hum Mut 2: 317

Levran O, Desnick RJ, Schuchman EH. 1991b. Niemann-Pick type B disease. Identification of a single codon deletion in the acid sphingomyelinase gene and genotype/phenotype correlations in type A and B patients. J ClinInvest 88: 806

Millard EE, Gale SE, Dudley N, Zhang J, Schaffer JE, Ory DS. 2005. The sterol-sensing domain of the Niemann-Pick C1 (NPC1) protein regulates trafficking of low density lipoprotein cholesterol. J Biol Chem 280: 28581

Millat G, Chikh K, Naureckiene S, Sleat DE, Fensom AH, Higaki K, Elleder M, Lobel P, Vanier MT. 2001a. Niemann-Pick disease type C: spectrum of HE1 mutations and genotype/phenotype correlations in the NPC2 group. Am J Hum Genet 69: 1013

Millat G, Marçais C, Tomasetto C, Chikh K, Fensom AH, Harzer K, Wenger DA, Ohno K, Vanier MT. 2001b. Niemann-Pick C1 disease: correlations between NPC1 mutations, levels of NPC1 protein, and phenotypes emphasize the functional significance of the putative sterol-sensing domain and of the cysteine-rich luminal loop. Am J Hum Genet 68: 1373

Millat G, Marçais C, Rafi MA, Yamamoto T, Morris JA, Pentchev PG, Ohno K, Wenger DA, Vanier MT. 1999. Niemann-Pick C1 disease: the I1061T substitution is a frequent mutant allele in patients of Western European descent and correlates with a classic juvenile phenotype. Am J Hum Genet 65: 1321

Naureckiene S, Sleat DE, Lackland H, Fensom A, Vanier MT, Wattiaux R, Jadot M, Lobel P. 2000. Identification of HE1 as the second gene of Niemann-Pick C disease. Science 290: 2298

Patterson MC, Vanier MT, Suzuki K, Morris JA, Carstea E, Neufeld EB, Blanchette-Mackie JE, Pentchev P. 2001. Niemann-Pick Disease type C: a lipid trafficking disorder. In: Scriver CR, Beaudet AL, Sly WS, Valle D, editors. The metabolic and molecular bases of inherited disease. New York: McGraw Hill. p 3611–3634

Patterson MC, Hendriksz CJ, Walterfang M, Sedel F, Vanier MT, Wijburg F, Group N-CGW. 2012. Recommendations for the diagnosis and management of Niemann-Pick disease type C: an update. Mol Genet Metab 106: 330

Pentchev PG, Comly ME, Kruth HS, Tokoro T, Butler J, Sokol J, Filling-Katz M, Quirk JM, Marshall DC, Patel S, et al. 1987. Group C Niemann-Pick disease: faulty regulation of low-density lipoprotein uptake and cholesterol storage in cultured fibroblasts. FASEB J 1: 40

Quintern LE, Schuchman EH, Levran O, Suchi M, Ferlinz K, Reinke H, Sandhoff K, Desnick RJ. 1989. Isolation of cDNA clones encoding human acid-sphingomyelinase: Occurrence of alternatively processed transcripts. EMBO J 8: 2469

Ribeiro I, Marcão A, Amaral O, Sá Miranda MC, Vanier MT, Millat G. 2001. Niemann-Pick type C disease: NPC1 mutations associated with severe and mild cellular cholesterol trafficking alterations. Hum Genet 109: 24

Runz H, Dolle D, Schlitter AM, Zschocke J. 2008. NPC-db, a Niemann-Pick type C disease gene variation database. Hum Mutat 29: 345

Schneider PB, Kennedy EP. 1967. Sphingomyelinase in normal human spleens and in spleens from subjects with Niemann-Pick disease. J Lipid Res 8: 202

Schuchman EH, Suchi M, Takahashi T, Sandhoff K, Desnick RJ. 1991. Human acid sphingomyelinase: Isolation, nucleotide sequence, and expression of the full-length and alternatively spliced cDNA. Biol Chem 266: 8531

Schuchman EH, Levran O, Pereira LV, Desnick RJ. 1992. Structural organization and complete nucleotide sequence of the gene encoding human acid sphingomyelinase (SMPD1). Genomics 12: 1

Schuchman EH, Desnick RJ. 2001. Niemann-Pick disease types A and B: acid sphingomyelinase deficiencies. In: The metabolic and molecular bases of inherited disease. (Scriver et al., eds.) New York: McGraw Hill. 3589

Seker Yilmaz B, Baruteau J, Rahim AA, Gissen P. 2020. Clinical and Molecular Features of Early Infantile Niemann Pick Type C Disease. Int J Mol Sci 21: 5059

Siegmund H. 1921. Lipoidzellhyperplasie der Milz und Splenomegalie Gaucher. Verh Dtsch Pathol Ges 18: 59

Simonaro CM, Desnick RJ, McGovern MM, Wasserstein MP, Schuchman EH. 2002. The demographics and distribution of Type B Niemann-Pick disease: novel mutations lead to new genotype/phenotype correlations. Am J Hum Genet 71: 1413

Simonaro CM, Park JH, Eliyahu E, Shtraizent N, Mc Govern MM, Schuchman EH. 2006. Imprinting at the SMPD1 locus: implications for acid sphingomyelinase-deficient Niemann-Pick disease. Am J Hum Genet 78: 865

Storch J, Xu Z. 2009. Niemann-Pick C2 (NPC2) and intracellular cholesterol trafficking. Biochim Biophys Acta 1791: 671

Vanier MT, Ferlinz K, Rousson R, Duthel S, Louisot P, Sandhoff K, Suzuki K. 1993. Deletion of arginine (608) in acid sphingomyelinase is the prevalent mutation among Niemann-Pick disease type B patients from Northern Africa. Hum Genet 92: 325

Vanier MT, Millat G. 2003. Niemann-Pick disease type C. Clin Genet 64: 269

Vanier MT, Gissen P, Bauer P, Coll MJ, Burlina A, Hendriksz CJ, Latour P, Goizet C, Welford RW, Marquardt T, Kolb SA. 2016. Diagnostic tests for Niemann-Pick disease type C (NP-C): A critical review. Mol Genet Metab 118: 244

Wassif CA, Cross JL, Iben J, Sanchez-Pulido L, Cougnoux A, Platt FM, Ory DS, Ponting CP, Bailey-Wilson JE, Biesecker LG, Porter FD. 2016. High incidence of unrecognized visceral/neurological late-onset Niemann-Pick disease, type C1, predicted by analysis of massively parallel sequencing data sets. Genet Med 18: 41

Xu Y, Zhang Q, Tan L, Xie X, Zhao Y. 2019. The characteristics and biological significance of NPC2: Mutation and disease. Mutat Res 782: 108284

Zampieri S, Filocamo M, Pianta A, Lualdi S, Gort L, Coll MJ, Sinnott R, Geberhiwot T, Bembi B, Dardis A. 2016. SMPD1 Mutation Update: Database and Comprehensive Analysis of Published and Novel Variants. Hum Mutat 37: 139

Zhang H, Wang Y, Gong Z, Li X, Qiu W, Han L, Ye J, Gu X. 2013. Identification of a distinct mutation spectrum in the SMPD1 gene of Chinese patients with acid sphingomyelinase-deficient Niemann-Pick disease. Orphanet J Rare Dis 8: 15

Zhou YF, Metcalf MC, Garman SC, Edmunds T, Qiu H, Wei RR. 2016. Human acid sphingomyelinase structures provide insight to molecular basis of Niemann-Pick disease. Nat Commun 7: 13082

Diagnosis of Niemann-Pick disease type C (NPC)

4. Diagnosis of Niemann-Pick disease type C (NPC)

Niemann-Pick disease type C (NPC) is a rare neurovisceral lysosomal disorder caused by autosomal recessive mutations in NPC1 or NPC2 (95% and 4% of patients, respectively).

- The diagnosis is not easy and requires specialist knowledge. There is no simple laboratory enzymatic test to prove a lack of NPC1 or NPC2.
- The clinical suspicion is sometimes vague as long as characteristic key findings are not recognized.
- Laboratory diagnostics are complex and the disease is not well known due to its rarity. Reliable figures on the frequency, incidence and prevalence of NPC are not available in Germany.

The analysis of four independent exome sequencing databases in the USA resulted in a conservatively estimated incidence of 1/92,104 for NPC1 and 1/2,858,998 for NPC2, which matches the clinical data from the USA and France quite well (Wassif et al. 2016).

According to epidemiological calculations for the prevalence of the two most common NPC1 variants in the USA, the frequency for late-onset forms was estimated at 1/19,000 to 1/36,000. This suggests that previous prevalence estimates may be too low and that the adult form (these two NPC1 variants are most likely to cause juvenile and adult forms) is significantly underdiagnosed. The diagnosis of NPC is usually made on average 4.1 years after the onset of neurological symptoms. Late diagnosis narrows the therapeutic window.

The first international recommendations for the clinical management and diagnosis of NPC were drawn up in 2009 (Group et al. 2009) on the basis of a literature review and the consensus of an expert panel. They were renewed in 2012 after a second meeting of the working group (Patterson et al. 2012). Intermediate progress in the field of NPC screening technologies with biomarkers and molecular genetic diagnostic methods then justified an update of these recommendations in 2017 (Patterson et al. 2017). The development and availability of fast and reliable biomarkers (oxysterols, lysosphingomyelin derivatives and bile acids) has significantly simplified and improved the detection of patients with NPC in recent years. In addition, the increasing availability of next-generation sequencing techniques (NGS, e.g. phenotype-specific gene panels) has improved diagnostic possibilities. The use of genetic tests in clinical practice, especially with risk cohorts that are characterized by a key finding (e.g. ataxia, neonatal cholestatic hepatopathy) has led to a diagnosis in many cases. Earlier recommendations regarding genetic diagnosis focused on the identification of individual patients with a high clinical suspicion of NPC (Patterson et al. 2017).

4.1. Recommendations for differential diagnosis and initial diagnosis

General principles

- All patients suspected of having NPC require an accurate and detailed clinical examination.
- The diagnostic process should be carried out at regional or national centers that are specialized in hereditary metabolic disorders and have experience with NPC.
- Visceral, neurologic, ophthalmic, and psychiatric manifestations should be recorded and tracked.

Current state of knowledge regarding psychiatric assessment (Bonnot et al. 2019a, 2019b)

- Psychiatric symptoms and cognitive disorders were observed in 45% and 61%, respectively, in the evaluation at the time of diagnosis. **Almost all patients develop psychiatric symptoms during the course of the disease.**
- However, no specific neuropsychiatric profile was identified.
- Patients with NPC, especially adults, can experience a variety of psychiatric symptoms, the most common being cognitive impairment (decreased executive function, memory, and psychomotor speed), schizophrenia, and other symptoms including depression.
- These symptoms can superimpose other symptoms of NPC.

- Due to the inherent difficulties in examining patients in psychiatric practice, undiagnosed patients should be expected in this setting.

Assessment of ocular motor function (Bremova-Ertl et al. 2021)

- Eye movements (saccades, gaze tracking, gaze hold function, optokinetic nystagmus should be examined (neurocular.com).
- Impaired vertical saccades, commonly referred to as vertical supranuclear gaze palsy (VSGP) – but correctly termed as vertical supranuclear saccade palsy (VSSP) – are of particular concern in NPC as they are an early sign of disease.
- VSSP is characteristic of NPC. There are hardly any differential diagnoses, especially in childhood and adolescence, but also in young adulthood.
- Slow and hypometric vertical saccades are often masked by blinking. This blinking when looking up or down may be noticeable when observing the patient.
- The patients often tilt their head backwards to look up. As this head position gives the impression that the patients are looking under something this sign and behavior is called "underlooking".

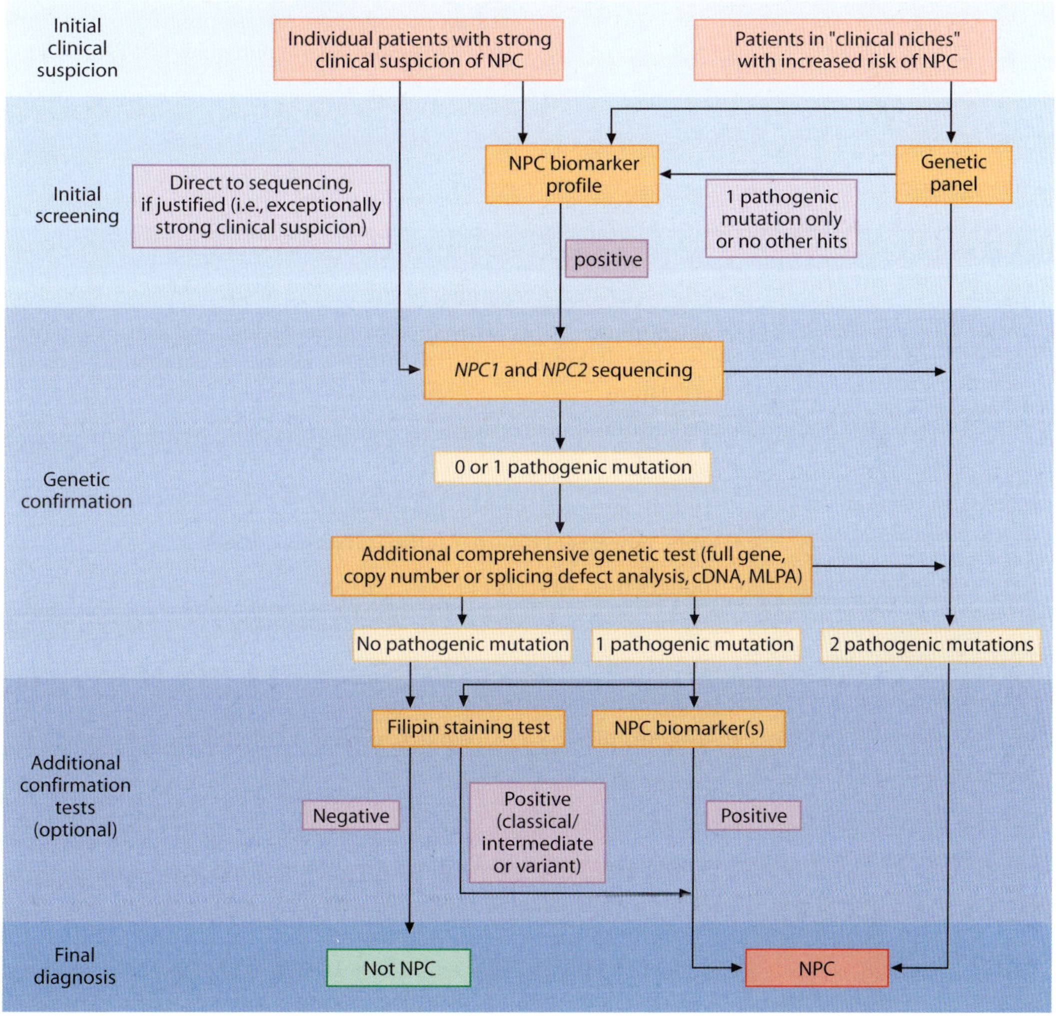

Figure 4.1: Diagnostic algorithm for the use of biomarkers and genetic testing in Niemann-Pick disease type C (NPC). Modified after Patterson et al. 2017.

- As the disease progresses, VSSP appears. This is typically followed by impairment of the horizontal saccades and then horizontal supranuclear palsy.
- Video oculography enables the recording of all types of eye movements and can be used for quantitative analysis of eye motor skills (eyeseecam.com/).
- VSSP can be present before visceral, neurological or psychiatric manifestations and is sometimes the only symptom of NPC in adults.

Vertical supranuclear saccade palsy (VSSP) is a sensitive and specific sign for NPC.

4.2. Clinical diagnosis and key findings in NPC

4.2.1. Neuropsychological diagnosis and key findings

The cognitive deficits in NPC impair everyday function and quality of life. Early diagnosis could identify cognitive deficits. Cognitive interventions and support measures can have a positive influence on the course of the disease. Treatment of NPC disease should be based on a multidisciplinary approach to manage symptoms, maintain neurological function, and ensure the best possible quality of life. Early detection of the neurological and psychological symptoms of the disease is necessary to reduce neurological disease progression and improve patient care and outcomes (☞ Table 4.1).

Clinical picture	Clinical signs that should be noted
Ataxia	• early-onset ataxia beginning before the age of 40 • "ataxia plus": VSSP, dystonia; cognitive decline; atypical psychiatric disorders; Babinski reflex rather than true spastic paraparesis; mental retardation • ataxia without neuropathy • ataxia of unknown etiology
Intellectual retardation and developmental delay	• visceral signs, e.g. (hepato)splenomegaly • subtle movement disorder (ataxia/dystonia), VSSP
Cognitive impairment and premature cognitive decline	• younger than 40 years old • neurological signs (e.g. ataxia, VSSP, dystonia)
Dystonia	• generalized dystonia • younger than 40 years old • "dystonia plus": VSSP, cognitive decline or psychiatric disorders
Frontotemporal dementia	• younger than 40 years old
Atypical schizophrenia/ early-onset psychosis	• resistance to treatment • neurological signs (e.g. ataxia, VSSP, dystonia) • organic characteristics: visual hallucinations, comorbid cognitive impairment
Visceral symptoms in children	• isolated infantile splenomegaly or cholestasis or hepatosplenomegaly or fetal/neonatal ascites and neurological signs (e.g. ataxia, VSSP, dystonia)

Table 4.1: Clinical patient groups at increased risk for NPC. Modified after Patterson et al. 2017.

4.2.2. Laboratory diagnostics and biomarkers

A reliable blood or urine test is a prerequisite for diagnosing an ultra-rare disease. For this purpose, substances that normally do not occur or only occur in low concentrations (called biomarkers) have to accumulate in a body fluid as a result of the disease and a reliable test is required to detect them. Ideally, there should be no area of overlap between healthy and sick people.

For decades such a test for NPC disease was not available; useful tests were only developed in recent years. The absence of such a test resulted in massive underdiagnosis of the disease and often decades of delay in diagnosis. The path to diagnosis in such a rare disease is often marked by wrong turns, and the first suspected diagnosis is not always the right one. When there is no simple laboratory test, but rather a tissue sample with subsequent cell culture is necessary for diagnosis, the consequence is that the examination is either not carried out at all or late in the diagnostic procedure.

The development of simple blood tests to diagnose NPC disease was a diagnostic revolution and has made the process so much easier that significantly more patients have been found in the past 10 years than ever before. Nevertheless, there are still patients today who wait decades between the onset of symptoms and diagnosis, so that the urgent appeal to the reader of these lines is made to use the new blood tests as generously as possible. The symptoms of the disease are usually irreversible, but the disease is treatable. A delay in diagnosis leads to irreversible, avoidable or at least delayable damage.

After the blood tests were initially very susceptible to interference and were reserved for a few special laboratories worldwide, very robust biomarker assays were developed that also work with dried blood spot cards. As a result, a vision of many NPC specialists is within reach – that one day affected children can be discovered by a newborn screening test and the disease will be perfectly treatable so the development of symptoms can be avoided. Although NPC disease is still fatal in all cases, this goal has become realistic thanks to the increasing improvement in drug therapy.

A large number of diagnostically usable biomarkers with different advantages and disadvantages are now available. It is largely irrelevant which biomarker is used. All of them allow a reliable diagnosis in the hands of an experienced laboratory. The choice of the biomarker by the individual health care provider should depend less on theoretical considerations than on the local availability of the test.

At the time of writing, the laboratory of the authors of this article is offering a free biomarker determination as part of a scientific research project (www.npc-test.com, one-time registration required).

Historical review

Until recently, the gold standard for diagnosing NPC disease was the so-called filipin test. Filipin is a cyclic fluorescent dye that specifically binds to cholesterol in tissue or cell cultures, which can then be detected.

Since NPC disease is based on intracellular sequestration and transport disruption of cholesterol, which accumulates in endosomes, cells from NPC sufferers have significantly more intense cholesterol staining than those of healthy individuals. The test is very reliable, but only few specialised laboratories in the world have the required experience. The main disadvantage, however, is that a skin biopsy must first be made to carry out the test. The fibroblasts have to be cultured from the skin biopsy, which in turn requires a cell culture laboratory and takes about 4-6 weeks. Then one of the few special laboratories that offer the test has to be found. The filipin test has therefore become obsolete today, apart from a few special cases. The same applies to the detection of storage cells in the bone marrow.

In the past, the activity of chitotriosidase in plasma was often used as a biomarker for NPC. Chitotriosidase is an enzyme that is mainly found in macrophages. Storage processes in these cells, but also inflammation-related cell activation, can lead to an increased production of chitotriosidase in these cells and to an increased blood concentration. This method is established in many laboratories, but is not specific for NPC, as the activity of chitotriosidase is also increased in other lysosomal diseases, e.g. Gaucher disease. This can also be the case in inflammatory diseases such as histiocytosis. In addition, there is a frequent duplication in the *CHIT1* gene, which leads to a complete loss of chitotriosidase activity. At around 6%, this affects a relevant part of the population in a homozygous form. In this case, chitotriosidase activity cannot be used as a biomarker, since no increased chitotriosidase activity can occur even if the disease is present. Another limitation is the fact that adult patients often show no or only a borderline increase in chitotriosidase.

Modern biomarkers

The heterogeneous phenotype and unspecific symptoms in Niemann-Pick type C represent a major diagnostic challenge for the treating physician. For a long time there was no specific biomarker for NPC. However, over the past few years great advances have been made in the field of selective screening and diagnosis of Niemann-Pick type C. Sensitive and specific biomarkers are now available that can be detected in a simple blood test and make diagnosis much easier. Two main biochemical markers are currently used in everyday clinical practice: cholestantriol and Lyso-SM-509. Other biomarkers are still being developed or are only offered in a few laboratories.

Oxysterols

So-called oxysterols (cholesterol oxidation products) were described as the first promising biomarkers for NPC in 2010 (Porter et al. 2010). The disruption of cholesterol transport leads to increased non-enzymatic oxidation of a very small part of the accumulated cholesterol in NPC cells (☞ Figure 4.2).

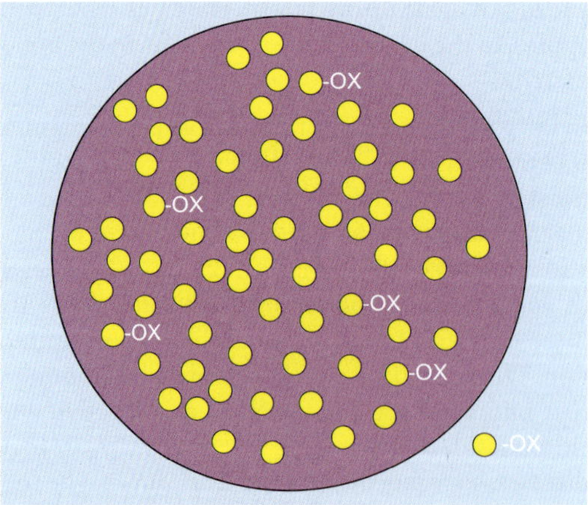

Figure 4.2: Cholesterol (yellow) is absorbed into the cell via the LDL receptor and then reaches the endosome (purple), where receptor and cholesterol are separated from one another in an acidic environment and the latter is bound by the NPC1 and NPC2 proteins after desterification. A lack of either protein leads to an accumulation of cholesterol in the organelle. A small part of the accumulating cholesterol is subject to non-enzymatic oxidation (●-OX) and can be used as a biomarker.

These oxidation products of cholesterol can be detected in the plasma by gas chromatography-mass spectrometry (GC-MS) or liquid chromatography-mass spectrometry (LC-MS/MS). It was shown that especially 7-ketocholesterol (7-KC) and cholestane-3β,5α,6β-triol (C-triol) are increased in the plasma of NPC1 and NPC2 patients (Boenzi et al. 2014; Jiang et al. 2011; Porter et al. 2010; Reunert et al. 2015; ☞ Figure 4.3).

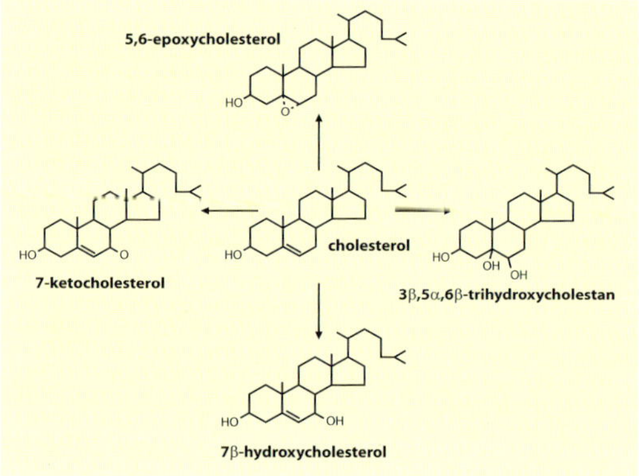

Figure 4.3: The accumulating cholesterol (middle) receives a keto group (7-KC, left) by oxidation or 2 further and thus a total of 3 hydroxyl groups (C-triol, right) by oxidative cleavage of the double bond.

The preferred oxysterol biomarker is C-triol, as it has a higher sensitivity and specificity compared to 7-KC (Boenzi et al. 2016). For several years, the clinical use of cholestanetriol was tested on samples from patients with suspected Niemann-Pick type C (Reunert et al. 2016). All positive samples were subjected to genetic analysis. More than 100 patients with mutations in NPC1 and 4 patients with mutations in NPC2 could thus be helped to a rapid diagnosis (Figure ☞ 4.4).

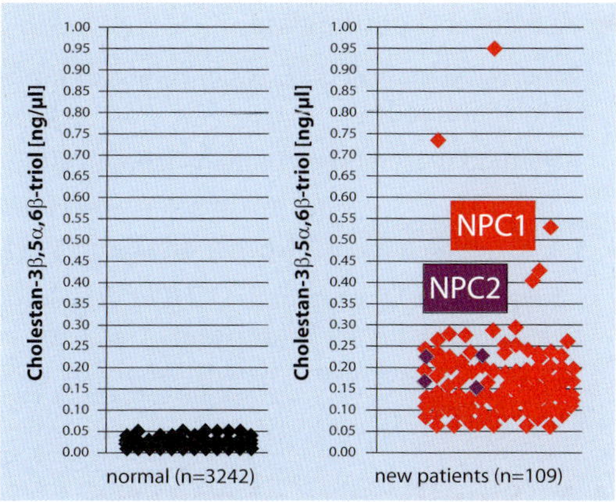

Figure 4.4: In the selective screening of a good 3,200 samples, more than 100 new NPC patients were detected by oxysterol test in 5 years, many times more than in the years before introduction of the biomarker test.

As a secondary finding, it turned out that increased C-triol concentrations occur not only in Niemann-Pick type C, but also in other related diseases, e.g. Niemann-Pick type A/B (NPA/B) and LAL deficiency (lysosomal acid lipase deficiency).

A weak point of the oxysterols is the poor stability of the sample at room temperature. Longer storage of the samples (>72 hours) at room temperature can lead to autoxidation of the cholesterol and thus to false positive results (Reunert et al. 2016). This means that the biomarker can only be used in countries where the infrastructure allows a short transport time to the specialised laboratory. In addition, the test may be false positive in a hemolytic blood sample. Heterozygous gene carriers can show elevated C-triol levels although they do not become ill themselves.

In newborns with cholestasis, oxysterols are increased in the absence of NPC disease and can only be used to a limited extent as the only biomarker for NPC (Polo et al. 2016).

The determination of the oxysterols requires an EDTA blood sample taken from a venous system; the biomarker cannot be determined from a dried blood spot card.

► Lyso-SM-509

The currently most widespread biomarker for Niemann-Pick type C is so-called Lyso-SM-509. It was first described as a lipid with an unknown structure (Giese et al. 2015). In 2019, the exact biochemical structure could finally be identified (Sidhu et al. 2019).

Lyso-SM-509 is an N-acyl-phosphocholine-serine, more precisely N-palmitoyl-O-phosphocholine-serine (PPCS). In most laboratories, however, the name Lyso-SM-509 is currently used. Plasma Lyso-SM-509 is elevated in both NPC and in NPA/B patients and appears to be more sensitive and reliable than C-triol. Another advantage is the stability even at room temperature and the possibility of analysis from dried blood spot cards as used in newborn screening. This enables easier sampling and uncomplicated shipping.

Lyso-sphingomyelin (Lyso-SM) is another lipid that is elevated in the plasma in NPC and NPA/B patients. In NPC, however, the increase in Lyso-SM is less than in NPA/B. A combination of different biomarkers such as C-triol, Lyso-SM-509 and Lyso-SM enables differentiation between NPC and NPA/B.

► Further biomarkers

In addition to C-triol, Lyso-SM-509 and Lyso-SM, some pathological bile acids are also elevated in patients with NPC because bile acids are made from cholesterol. The accumulation of oxysterols in the NPC cell means that oxidized cholesterol molecules are used as a building block for bile acid biosynthesis and thus chemically altered bile acids are produced.

The preferred analyte is 3β,5α,6β-trihydroxy-cholanoyl-glycine (Jiang et al. 2016; Mazzacuva et al. 2016). This can be detected in plasma and urine as well as in dried blood spot cards. In contrast to C-triol, pre-analytical auto-oxidation is not a problem. 3β,5α,6β-trihydroxy-cholanoyl-glycine also seems to be more specific for NPC than C-triol and differentiates NPC carriers from patients. However, it is also increased in patients with NPA/B. This assay is not yet established in many laboratories and is mostly not available in everyday clinical practice. A clear advantage is the possibility of diagnosing the disease from a urine sample, which e.g. in pediatrics or psychiatry further lowers the diagnostic inhibition threshold, since no blood sample has to be taken.

Recommendations for diagnosing Niemann-Pick type C

New guidelines consider the known biomarkers and recommend their measurement as the first diagnostic step (Patterson et al. 2017). Due to its invasive method, the filipin test is no longer recommended as a primary test, but can be used to confirm unexplained cases.

No biomarker is 100% sensitive and specific. However, available biomarkers achieve a sensitivity of more than 99%, i.e. almost every patient can be detected. The fact that related lysosomal storage diseases can also cause a positive test lowers the specificity somewhat. However, this does not have to be a disadvantage, as a positive biomarker test narrows the differential diagnosis down to a few diseases and, in case of doubt, will lead to the diagnosis of a different ultra-rare disease.

Any positive biomarker test should be confirmed by genetic testing. While the *NPC2* gene is small and quick to examine, the *NPC1* gene, with its 25 exons, is much more complex. The rapid drop in price for whole exome examinations means that more and more patients are found via a primary genetic test. Nevertheless, in these cases, the genetic findings should be validated by means of a biomarker test.

Summary of available biomarkers

▶ Oxysterols (cholesterol oxidation products)

+ best explored, widely recognized, accessible, widely used

± increased concentrations also occur in other diseases, including NPA/B and LAL deficiency (lysosomal acid lipase)

– poor stability of the sample at room temperature (autoxidation of cholesterol) and susceptibility to hemolysis

– also increased in newborns with cholestasis

▶ Lyso-sphingomyelin-509 (or N-palmitoyl-O-phosphocholine serine)

+ appears to be more sensitive and reliable than C-triol

+ stability even at room temperature

+ analysis also possible from dried blood spot cards

± increased in NPC and for NPA/B

▶ Activity of chitotriosidase

+ increased in most NPC patients (less or not at all in adulthood)

+ method is established in many laboratories

– unspecific, as it is also increased in other lysosomal diseases, e.g. in Gaucher disease

– frequent duplication in the *CHIT1* gene leads to a complete loss of chitotriosidase activity; in this case chitotriosidase activity cannot be used as a biomarker

4.3. Significance of genetic testing in NPC

Biomarkers alone are strong indicators of NPC, but the diagnosis must be confirmed by genetic testing. It is critically important to genetically confirm the diagnosis in patients with strong clinical suspicion and/or a biomarker profile consistent with NPC. Almost 700 variants, 400 of which are referred to as pathogenic mutations, are known for *NPC1* and approximately 25 have been described for *NPC2*. The highly polymorphic nature of *NPC1* can make diagnostic conclusions difficult and the interpretation of new mutations challenging. The estimated proportion of NPC cases in which the detection of mutations on both alleles can be achieved using routine sequencing methods (exons and accompanying sections) is currently more than 90%.

Some genetic changes such as large deletions/duplications or deep intronic changes cannot be reliably detected using traditional sequencing methods. The detection of such mutations (estimated 5% of the alleles) therefore requires different techniques. A small percentage of mutated *NPC1* alleles (less than 5%) has so far remained undetected in all experienced groups.

The two most commonly found *NPC1* mutations worldwide are p.I1061T, which accounts for 20% of the mutated alleles in Western Europeans, and p.P1007A, also in patients of European descent. A number of recurring mutations are common in patients from certain countries, such as Iran. Some *NPC1* mutations (including p.P1007A) are associated with less pronounced changes in cholesterol transport. Some missense mutations seem to be clearly related to a late-onset form of NPC, even in

<table>
<tr><th></th><th>Infantile neurovisceral ASMD (NPA)</th><th>Chronic neurovisceral ASMD (intermediary, NPA/B)</th><th>Chronic visceral ASMD (NPB)</th></tr>
<tr><td>Initial manifestation, life expectancy, and common genotypes</td><td>• initial manifestation in infancy
• onset of death at 3 years of age (median 27 months)
• associated with p.R498L-, p.L304P- and p.P333Sfs*52 variants</td><td>• initial manifestation in childhood
• death as a result of liver and lung involvement, time of death can vary from childhood to adulthood
• associated with p.Q294K- and p.W393G variants</td><td>• initial manifestation in childhood/adulthood
• usually survival into adulthood, progressive liver and lung disease can in some cases lead to earlier death
• associated with p.ΔR610-, p.P323A-, p.P330R and p.W393G variants</td></tr>
<tr><td>CNS</td><td>• short period of normal development followed by loss of acquired skills
• mild hypotension, loss of deep tendon reflexes, dysphagia</td><td>• slow progression of mild neurological symptoms after a period of normal development that can last 2 to 7 years
• peripheral neuropathy, extrapyramidal symptoms, psychiatric symptoms, learning disabilities
• ataxia beginning in early childhood</td><td>• no signs of neurodegeneration</td></tr>
<tr><td>Eyes</td><td>• ocular cherry red spot</td><td>• ocular cherry red spot or macula halo syndrome (☞ Figure 5.4)</td><td>• eye anomalies as an indication of neuronal storage, observed in some patients even without neurological disease</td></tr>
<tr><td>Gastrointestinal tract</td><td>• hepatosplenomegaly usually after 3 months (possibly massive)
• cholestatic jaundice
• feeding difficulties
• vomiting</td><td colspan="2">• hepatosplenomegaly
• splenomegaly usually precedes hepatomegaly
• mostly liver fibrosis
• portal hypertension
• abnormal results in liver function tests
• diarrhea</td></tr>
<tr><td>Respiratory tract</td><td>• interstitial lung disease
• frequent, recurrent respiratory infections, aspiration pneumonia</td><td colspan="2">• interstitial lung disease on imaging
• radiological findings can be very noticeable with no apparent symptoms
• limited significance of lung function tests</td></tr>
<tr><td>Heart</td><td>• no cardiac symptoms</td><td colspan="2">• heart valve disease
• mixed dyslipidemia with low HDL cholesterol
• early onset coronary heart disease</td></tr>
<tr><td>Musculoskeletal system</td><td>• no skeletal manifestation</td><td colspan="2">• bone and joint pain
• reduced bone density and pathological fractures
• delayed bone maturation
• growth restriction in childhood</td></tr>
<tr><td>Blood</td><td>• no hematological symptoms or mild thrombocytopenia</td><td colspan="2">• thrombocytopenia with bleeding tendency</td></tr>
<tr><td>Other</td><td>• sleep disorders
• irritability</td><td colspan="2">• headache
• recurrent ear infections</td></tr>
</table>

Table 4.2: Clinical features and natural course of ASMD phenotypes. Modified after McGovern MM et al. 2017.

compound heterozygosity with a very severe/null allele.

Approximately 25 disease-causing mutations (including one large deletion) have been described in the *NPC2* gene. Most of these are severe and result in a truncated protein and null alleles, but a few (p.V39M and p.P120S) result in later onset forms.

4.3.1. Next-generation sequencing (NGS) and gene panels

Sanger sequencing of genomic DNA (gDNA) or complementary DNA (cDNA) has traditionally been recommended in parallel with the filipin staining test to confirm the diagnosis of NPC. NGS technologies provide accurate and sensitive methods for genetic analysis. It is crucial that only high quality reads and integrated software tools are used.

More and more targeted gene and multigene panels, including NPC1 and NPC2, with full exons and exon-intron boundaries, are used to screen clinical patient groups at increased risk for NPC (Synofzik et al. 2015). NPC1 and NPC2 are contained in several gene panels, including early onset ataxia, epilepsy, dystonia, infantile cholestasis, specific congenital metabolic disorders (lysosomal storage diseases), organic psychoses, early onset cognitive decline, hepatosplenomegaly, and developmental delay. New gene panels are under development.

The diagnostic yield appears to be highest in patients with early onset ataxia, where 1 to 2% of patients have NPC. Even in infants with cholestatic hepatopathy, NPC is regularly diagnosed.

4.3.2. Differentiation from acid sphingomyelinase deficiency (ASMD)

Acid sphingomyelinase (ASMD) deficiency, commonly known as Niemann-Pick disease types A and B with intermediate forms, is a rare, progressive, and often fatal lysosomal storage disease (LSD). The prevalence at birth is estimated at 0.4-0.6/100,000. Although type A ASMD is more com-

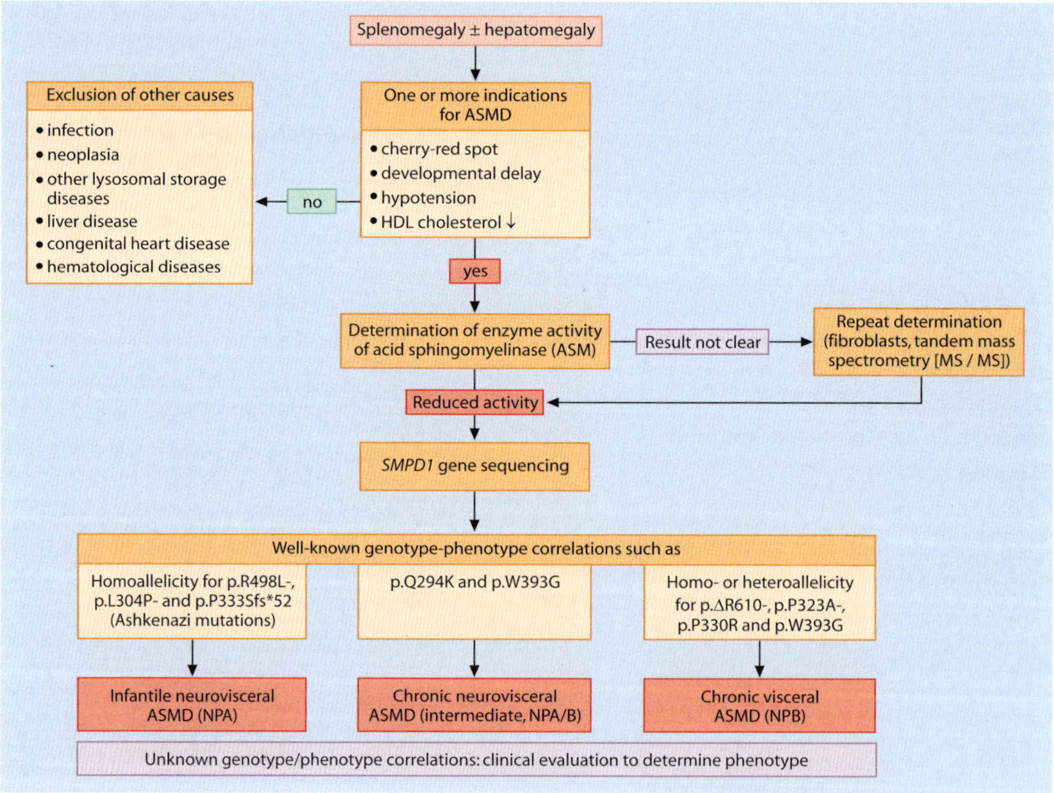

Figure 4.5: Algorithm for the differential diagnosis of ASMD in infancy and childhood. Modified after McGovern MM et al. 2017.

mon among people of Azkenazi Jewish descent, the three forms of ASMD are panethnic. ASMD was first described in 1914 and the genetic and biochemical basis as well as the clinical picture are different from NPC.

Although all patients with ASMD have the same basic metabolic defect, there is a wide diversity of clinical differences in the severity of the disease, which contribute to diagnostic challenges (☞ Table 4.2 and Figure 4.5). The severity of ASMD ranges from rapidly progressing neurovisceral disease in childhood, which is consistently fatal in early childhood, to slowly progressing chronic neurovisceral and chronic visceral forms. The remaining enzyme activity largely determines the extent of neurological involvement and the speed at which the disease progresses.

Due to the methodology used, the enzyme activity in routine diagnostics does not sufficiently reflect the remaining *in vivo* activity in the patient.

McGovern and colleagues reached agreement that if ASMD is suspected, an enzyme test for ASM activity should always be performed first. Gene sequencing should follow once the biochemical diagnosis is confirmed. Simultaneous determination of glucocerebrosidase activity is recommended to distinguish ASMD from Gaucher disease (Mc Govern et al. 2017).

Gene sequencing can be diagnostic if two pathogenic mutations are detected. However, the detection of a lack of enzyme activity remains the evidence of the presence of the disease, especially in view of the many unique mutations or genetic variants of unknown significance.

The results of other clinical and laboratory tests such as the presence of characteristic lipid-overloaded foam cells in the liver, spleen, airways and bone marrow, as well as low platelet counts and mixed dyslipidemia (low HDL cholesterol with high levels of LDL cholesterol and triglycerides) may very likely indicate an ASMS. However, they are not a substitute for the need for confirmatory enzyme test results.

The enzyme activity has traditionally been determined fluorometrically in leukocytes and fibroblasts. However, the laboratory implementation and interpretation is prone to errors. The quality of the available substrates is unsatisfactory. For a few

Symptoms	LALD	Gaucher disease	ASMD	NPC
CNS	–	–	–	ataxia, dysarthria, cognitive decline[2]
Slowed and hypometric saccades	–	± horizontal (GD3)	–	+ (vertical)[2]
Lung	–	±	++	±
Liver	steatosis, fibrosis, cirrhosis	mild to severe hepatomegaly	fibrosis	cholestatic liver
Spleen	not involved to ++	+++	+++	+ to ++
Chitotriosidase (nmol/mL/h)	500-2,000	+++	1,000-4,000	normal to 1,500
Cholesterol	+ to ++[1]	LDL-C ↓ to normal	+ to ++	unchanged to +
Triglycerides	+[1]	normal	+	unchanged
HDL cholesterol	↓↓[1]	normal	↓↓	↓
Lyso-sphingolipids	-	lyso-GL1 +++	lyso-SM +++ lyso-SM-509 +++	lyso-SM + lyso-SM-509 +++

Table 4.3: Differential diagnostic aspects in lysosomal acid lipase deficiency (**LALD**), Gaucher disease, acid sphingomyelinase deficiency (**ASMD**) and Niemann-Pick disease type C (**NPC**). **GD3** = Gaucher disease type 3, ↓ = lowered, ↓↓ = significantly lowered, + = increased , ++ = significantly increased, +++ = very significantly increased, ± = partly increased, partly not, **LDL-C** = low-density lipoprotein cholesterol. Modified after Valayannopoulos et al. 2017.

[1] not in patients with early childhood disease

[2] in the later course of the disease

years now, tandem mass spectrometry (MS/MS) has been available as a new method that is preferably used in dried blood spot testing (DBS). The analysis in the DBS is fast and superior to conventional tests in terms of informative value and laboratory effort.

Comparisons with fluorimetry have shown that a better distinction between unaffected and affected persons is possible. Fluorometric substrates for acid sphingomyelinase measurement often lead to false negative results. In the case of the mutation p.Q294K, which is common in Eastern and Central Europe, the measurement results can even show an unusually high level of activity.

In addition to better substrate specificity and the elimination of radiochemicals, tandem mass spectrometry enables a multiplex measurement of enzyme activities that are included in the differential diagnosis of ASMD.

Diagnostic biomarkers for ASMD

Plasma chitotriosidase, a biomarker for macrophage activation, is significantly increased in several LSDs, including Gaucher disease and ASMD (Ries et al. 2006). In Gaucher disease, chitotriosidase is a useful parameter for the severity of disease and for monitoring the course of enzyme replacement therapy. Although the levels seen in ASMD are not as high as in patients with Gaucher disease, chitotriosidase can serve as a useful biomarker for ASMD. However, up to 6% of people have a recessively inherited chitotriosidase deficiency, and another 30% are carriers of the variant. The former do not express any enzyme activity, the carriers have a significantly lower activity.

The rarely used CCL18 plasma level is elevated in both Gaucher disease and ASMD. This marker is of particular use when patients are chitotriosidase deficient.

▶ Lyso-sphingomyelin (lyso-SM)

A reliable, meaningful and easy-to-determine biomarker is urgently needed for the diagnosis and treatment of acid sphingomyelinase deficiency (ASMD, also known as Niemann Pick A, A/B and B). Lyso-sphingomyelin (lyso-SM) appears to be a valuable candidate in this regard. A broad application in clinical routine will significantly improve and simplify diagnosis. A recently published study found a relationship between lyso-SM levels and clinical subtype or severity. Future studies are needed to determine how these values correlate with response to treatment. A therapeutic biomarker would then also be available for ASMD (Breilyn et al. 2021, Kuchar et al. 2017).

4.4. Differential diagnosis of similar lysosomal diseases

ASMD, NPC, LALD and Gaucher disease are storage diseases that can be conspicuous with very similar findings and symptoms. Table 4.3 provides help with differential diagnosis.

References

Boenzi S, Deodato F, Taurisano R, Martinelli D, Verrigni D, Carrozzo R, Bertini E, Pastore A, Dionisi-Vici C, and Johnson DW. A new simple and rapid LC–ESI-MS/MS method for quantification of plasma oxysterols as dimethylaminobutyrate esters. Its successful use for the diagnosis of Niemann–Pick type C disease. Clin Chim Acta 2014;437: 93-100.

Boenzi S, Deodato F, Taurisano R, Goffredo BM, Rizzo C, and Dionisi-Vici C. Evaluation of plasma cholestane-3β,5α,6β-triol and 7-ketocholesterol in inherited disorders related to cholesterol metabolism. J Lipid Res 2016; 57: 361-367.

Bonnot O, Klunemann HH, Velten C, Torres Martin JV, and Walterfang M. Systematic review of psychiatric signs in Niemann-Pick disease type C. World J Biol Psychiatry 2019a;20(4):320-32.

Bonnot O, Gama CS, Mengel E, Pineda M, Vanier MT, Watson L, et al. Psychiatric and neurological symptoms in patients with Niemann-Pick disease type C (NP-C): Findings from the International NPC Registry. World J Biol Psychiatry 2019b;20(4):310-9.

Breilyn MS, Zhang W, Yu C, and Wasserstein MP. Plasma lyso-sphingomyelin levels are positively associated with clinical severity in acid sphingomyelinase deficiency. Mol Genet Metab Rep 2021;28:100780.

Bremova-Ertl T, Abel L, Walterfang M, Salsano E, Ardissone A, Malinova V, et al. A cross-sectional, prospective ocular motor study in 72 patients with Niemann-Pick disease type C. Eur J Neurol 2021;28:3040-3050.

Giese AK, Mascher H, Grittner U, Eichler S, Kramp G, Lukas J, te Vruchte D, Al Eisa N, Cortina-Borja M, Porter FD, et al. A novel, highly sensitive and specific biomarker for Niemann-Pick type C1 disease. Orphanet J Rare Dis 2015;10: 78.

Group N-CGW, Wraith JE, Baumgartner MR, Bembi B, Covanis A, Levade T, et al. Recommendations on the diagnosis and management of Niemann-Pick disease type C. Mol Genet Metab 2009;98(1-2):152-65.

Jiang X, Sidhu R, Porter FD, Yanjanin NM, Speak AO, te Vruchte DT, et al. A sensitive and specific LC-MS/MS method for rapid diagnosis of Niemann-Pick C1 disease from human plasma. J Lipid Res 2011;52(7):1435-45.

Jiang X, Sidhu R, Mydock-McGrane L, Hsu FF, Covey DF, Scherrer DE, Earley B, Gale SE, Farhat NY, Porter FD, et al. Development of a bile acid-based newborn screen for Niemann-Pick disease type C. Sci Transl Med 2016;8: 337ra63.

Kuchar L, Sikora J, Gulinello ME, Poupetova H, Lugowska A, Malinova V, et al. Quantitation of plasmatic lysosphingomyelin and lysosphingomyelin-509 for differential screening of Niemann-Pick A/B and C diseases. Anal Biochem 2017;525:73-7.

Maekawa M, Jinnoh I, Matsumoto Y, Narita A, Mashima R, Takahashi H, et al. Structural Determination of Lysosphingomyelin-509 and Discovery of Novel Class Lipids from Patients with Niemann-Pick Disease Type C. Int J Mol Sci 2019;20(20).

Mazzacuva F, Mills P, Mills K, Camuzeaux S, Gissen P, Nicoli ER, Wassif C, Te Vruchte D, Porter FD, Maekawa M, et al. Identification of novel bile acids as biomarkers for the early diagnosis of Niemann-Pick C disease. FEBS Lett 2016;590: 1651-1662.

McGovern MM, Dionisi-Vici C, Giugliani R, Hwu P, Lidove O, Lukacs Z, Eugen Mengel K, Mistry PK, Schuchman EH, Wasserstein MP. 2017. Consensus recommendation for a diagnostic guideline for acid sphingomyelinase deficiency. Genet Med 19: 967-974

McGovern MM, Dionisi-Vici C, Giugliani R, Hwu P, Lidove O, Lukacs Z, et al. Consensus recommendation for a diagnostic guideline for acid sphingomyelinase deficiency. Genet Med 2017;19(9):967-74.

Patterson MC, Hendriksz CJ, Walterfang M, Sedel F, Vanier MT, Wijburg F, et al. Recommendations for the diagnosis and management of Niemann-Pick disease type C: an update. Mol Genet Metab 2012;106(3):330-44.

Patterson MC, Clayton P, Gissen P, Anheim M, Bauer P, Bonnot O, et al. Recommendations for the detection and diagnosis of Niemann-Pick disease type C: An update. Neurol Clin Pract 2017;7(6):499-511.

Patterson MC, Vecchio D, Prady H, Abel L, and Wraith JE. Miglustat for treatment of Niemann-Pick C disease: a randomised controlled study. Lancet Neurol 2007;6: 765-772.

Polo G, Burlina A, Furlan F, Kolamunnage T, Cananzi M, Giordano L, Zaninotto M, Plebani M, and Burlina A. High level of oxysterols in neonatal cholestasis: a pitfall in analysis of biochemical markers for Niemann-Pick type C disease. Clin Chem Lab Med 2016;CCLM 54.

Porter FD, Scherrer DE, Lanier MH, Langmade SJ, Molugu V, Gale SE, Olzeski D, Sidhu R, Dietzen DJ, Fu R, et al. Cholesterol oxidation products are sensitive and specific blood-based biomarkers for Niemann-Pick C1 disease. Sci Transl Med 2010;2: 56ra81.

Reunert J, Lotz-Havla AS, Polo G, Kannenberg F, Fobker M, Griese M, Mengel E, Muntau AC, Schnabel P, Sommerburg O, et al. Niemann-Pick Type C-2 Disease: Identification by Analysis of Plasma Cholestane-3β,5α,6β-Triol and Further Insight into the Clinical Phenotype. JIMD Rep 2015;23: 17-26.

Reunert J, Fobker M, Kannenberg F, Du Chesne I, Plate M, Wellhausen J, Rust S, and Marquardt T. Rapid Diagnosis of 83 Patients with Niemann Pick Type C Disease and Related Cholesterol Transport Disorders by Cholestantriol Screening. EBioMedicine 2016;4: 170-175.

Ries M, Schaefer E, Luhrs T, Mani L, Kuhn J, Vanier MT, et al. Critical assessment of chitotriosidase analysis in the rational laboratory diagnosis of children with Gaucher disease and Niemann-Pick disease type A/B and C. J Inherit Metab Dis 2006;29(5):647-52.

Sidhu R, Mondjinou Y, Qian M, Song H, Kumar AB, Hong X, Hsu FF, Dietzen DJ, Yanjanin NM, Porter FD, et al. *N* -acyl- *O* -phosphocholineserines: structures of a novel class of lipids that are biomarkers for Niemann-Pick C1 disease. J Lipid Res 2019;60: 1410-1424.

Synofzik M, Harmuth F, Stampfer M, Muller Vom Hagen J, Schols L, and Bauer P. NPC1 is enriched in unexplained early onset ataxia: a targeted high-throughput screening. J Neurol. 2015;262(11):2557-63.

Valayannopoulos V, Mengel E, Brassier A, Grabowski G. 2017. Lysosomal acid lipase deficiency: Expanding differential diagnosis. Mol Genet Metab 120: 62-66

Wassif CA, Cross JL, Iben J, Sanchez-Pulido L, Cougnoux A, Platt FM, et al. High incidence of unrecognized visceral/neurological late-onset Niemann-Pick disease, type C1, predicted by analysis of massively parallel sequencing data sets. Genet Med 2016;18(1):41-8.

Welford RW, Garzotti M, Marques Lourenco C, Mengel E, Marquardt T, Reunert J, et al. Plasma lysosphingomyelin demonstrates great potential as a diagnostic biomarker for Niemann-Pick disease type C in a retrospective study. PLoS One 2014;9(12):e114669.

Clinical manifestation

5. Clinical manifestation

5.1. Niemann-Pick disease type A and type B

Types A and B of Niemann-Pick disease reflect the two poles of the clinical spectrum of sphingomyelinase deficiency. The genetic defect and the resulting residual activity determine the clinical manifestations (Schuchman 2001). While little or no residual enzyme activity is measured in type A, significant residual activity in type B may prevent the onset of neurological symptoms. The clinical features of patients with sphingomyelinase deficiency, who cannot be assigned to either the classic type A or type B phenotype, have been poorly studied.

Phenotypic variability has led to categorization of subtypes based on severity and extent of neurologic involvement. In 2017, McGovern and colleagues proposed a standardized terminology for ASMD (acid sphingomyelinase deficiency) phenotypes to better describe the spectrum of the disease and to distinguish ASMD from Niemann-Pick type C of the same name.

Infantile neurovisceral ASMD (NPA)

This condition, also known as Niemann Pick type A disease, is the most severe form of ASMD. Patients have little to no residual ASM activity. Symptoms begin in early infancy with rapidly progressive systemic manifestations, including hepatosplenomegaly and lung involvement, neurodegeneration, hypotonia and failure to thrive. Psychomotor development may be normal for several months after birth before reaching a plateau at 6 to 15 months of age and then regressing. Death typically occurs before 3 years of age and often results from respiratory failure following infection.

Chronic neurovisceral ASMD

Also known as the intermediate form or Niemann-Pick type A/B disease, this form is characterized by slower progression of neurologic symptoms and longer survival compared to infantile neurovisceral ASMD. Ataxia, gross motor delays and learning disabilities are common. The progressive multisystemic disease manifestations are similar or more severe than in chronic visceral ASMD.

Chronic visceral ASMD

This form is also known as Niemann-Pick type B disease and is characterized by a variable age of onset, ranging from infancy to adulthood, and slowly progressive multisystemic disease manifestations without neurodegeneration. Patients may have a normal life expectancy or die prematurely from complications of the disease, which include respiratory failure, liver failure and/or hemorrhage. The most common initial diagnosis is hepatosplenomegaly in early childhood, although mild disease may not be diagnosed until adulthood. It is not uncommon for the spleen to be significantly enlarged (e.g., more than ten times normal). Common clinical features in childhood include delayed growth and puberty, fatigue, and bone and joint pain. Other findings include osteopenia and decreased platelet and white blood cell counts. Lung function may worsen over time, and interstitial lung disease and lung infections are common. A proatherogenic lipid profile (mixed dyslipidemia) is observed early in the course of the disease, and some patients develop coronary artery disease. The development of liver fibrosis, ranging from minimal fibrosis to cirrhosis, is common, and progression of liver disease contributes to early mortality in some patients. Progressive splenomegaly may result from portal hypertension.

The clinical manifestation and course of Niemann-Pick type A disease are relatively uniform. Pregnancy and birth are typically unremarkable. Occasionally, prolongated jaundice can be observed in the neonatal period. Usually, marked hepatosplenomegaly is noticed in the first 3 months of life, more rarely between the fourth and sixth month of life. Physical examination then also reveals moderate lymphadenopathy. Since hepatosplenomegaly and lymphadenopathy are usually suggestive of underlying malignancies, bone marrow aspiration is often performed for differential diagnosis. Bone marrow examination then reveals the characteristic Niemann-Pick foam cells. Microcytic anemia, which cannot always be treated by iron supplementation, and thrombocytopenia only appear in the further course of the disease (☞ Figure 5.1).

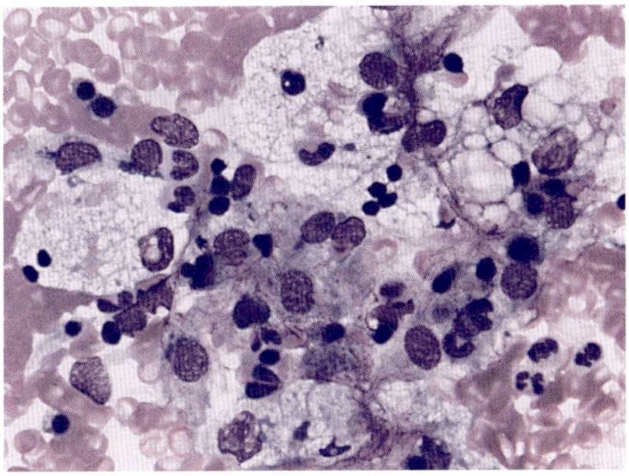

Figure 5.1: Accumulation of foam cells in the bone marrow.

The first neurological symptom is usually muscular hypotonia. Parents notice that the child is lagging behind peers in motor development and that there are increasing problems with feeding or breastfeeding.

Recurring vomiting and chronic constipation are common complications. Growth and weight gain now lag significantly behind peers. Bronchitis and aspiration pneumonia can complicate the course as early as 1 year of age. X-ray images show a fine-nodular, diffuse reticular interstitial pattern of lung disease (☞ Figure 5.2+5.3).

However, respiratory distress and pulmonary insufficiency are not the biggest problems in the first year of life for these patients. The bloated abdomen and in contrast thin, fragile appearance of the extremities are striking. The skin of patients with Niemann-Pick type A appears yellowish-brown or ochre in color. Xanthomas may be observed on the face or upper extremities. In contrast to Gaucher disease, bone involvement is mild despite comparable infiltration of storage cells. Presumably, other pathologic processes are involved in Gaucher disease. Osteoporosis due to physical inactivity and malnutrition is observed early.

At the age of 6 months, psychomotor retardation is evident in all patients. The further course of the disease shows progressive neurodegeneration. Muscular hypotonia increases and the children quickly lose their acquired skills (e.g. free sitting). Motor as well as mental abilities are equally affected by the neurodegenerative processes. In the final stage, the children have lost contact with their environment and persist in spasticity and rigidity. They usually die in the third year of life (Schuchman 2001).

In contrast to the rather stereotypical Niemann-Pick type A disease, the clinical manifestation and course of type B appear much more heterogeneous. In most patients, enlargement of the spleen and/or liver is noted in childhood, occasionally as early as infancy (Schuchman 2001). At the time of diagnosis, lung involvement in the form of a fine nodular, diffuse reticular interstitial pattern can almost always be detected radiologically. Occasionally, the diagnosis is not made until adulthood.

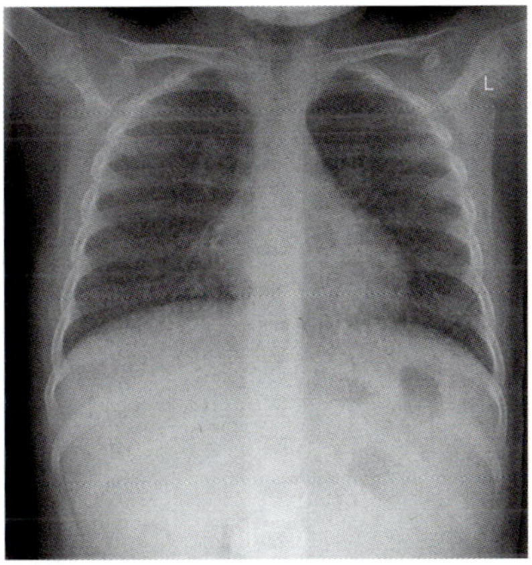

Figure 5.2: Diffuse reticular interstitial pattern in lung imaging of a 5-year-old girl with Niemann-Pick type B disease.

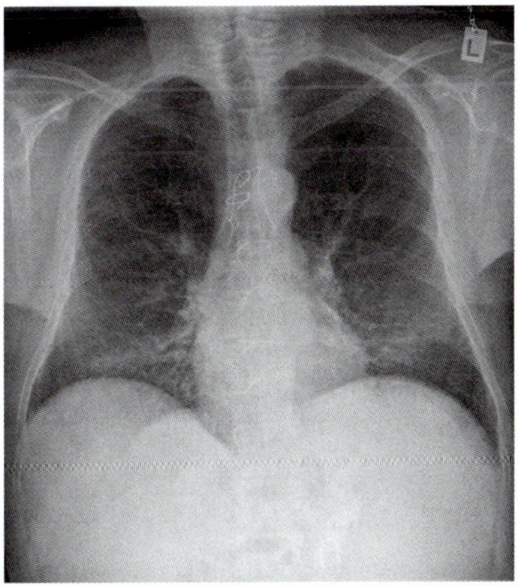

Figure 5.3: Diffuse reticular interstitial pattern of lung disease and hepatosplenomegaly in a 16-year-old patient with Niemann-Pick type B disease.

With increasing growth, hepatosplenomegaly is less noticeable. In some patients, spleen volume decreases (not only in relation to body weight but also the absolute size) in the second decade of life. Fibrotic remodeling processes probably play a role here.

Patients experience an impairment of quality of life due to increasing shortness of breath. Initially, patients notice exertional dyspnea and cyanosis caused by reduced oxygen diffusion due to alveolar infiltration. Severe bronchopneumonia with pulmonary insufficiency and cor pulmonale are feared, limiting complications (Minai et al. 2000). Concomitant hepatic insufficiency, marked by portal hypertension, ascites and coagulopathy, may further exacerbate the course (Takahashi et al. 1997).

At times, clinically relevant pancytopenia was treated by partial or complete splenectomy. Due to the small number of cases, no statement can be made about the effectiveness of this treatment.

In Niemann-Pick type A + B disease, most of the storage material can be found in the spleen. However, at least single foam cells are found in all tissues. The spleen is often enlarged more than tenfold (>1,000 cm³). It loses its soft consistency and oval, curved shape. The histologic architecture of the spleen is completely destroyed by infiltration of foam cells. In the most severe cases, the red pulp is completely substituted by foam cells.

The liver may also be significantly enlarged. A doubled liver volume indicates a storage fraction well in excess of 1,000 cm³. The liver is palpably harder than normal and shows a grayish-yellow color. In the early stages of storage, the sinuses are most commonly affected. As the disease progresses, the portal fields also become involved. In addition to the typical foam cells, large Kupffer cells and vacuolated parenchymal cells can be seen. The histologic architecture is highly variably altered. In advanced disease, the liver undergoes fibrotic remodeling. Liver cirrhosis represents the final stage (Schuchman 2001, Takahashi et al. 1997).

The lungs are usually affected early in the disease process in almost all patients, in contrast to Gaucher disease. The weight of the lung is significantly increased in Niemann-Pick A + B patients. Foam cells are found throughout the lung tissue as well as in arterial blood vessels and the lymphatic system. In advanced disease, significant amounts of foam cells are also found in the pulmonary alveoli and bronchial secretions. Inflammatory and fibrotic changes in the lungs are not usually among the characteristic histologic findings, although "sclerotic" alveolar septa and increased connective tissue around bronchi and vessels are occasionally seen (Minai et al. 2000, Schuchman 2001).

The bone marrow of affected patients generally appears hyperplastic. Up to 3% of the nuclear cells of the bone marrow may be foam cells. Foam cells in the bone marrow are usually larger than in the spleen, although phagocytosis of erythrocytes is less commonly found.

The extent of lymph node involvement is highly variable, with 3- to 5-fold enlarged lymph nodes frequently found. Lymphadenopathy is typically most pronounced mesenterically. However, tonsils and thymus gland may also be enlarged. Enlargements of peripheral lymph nodes are rarely observed. Similar to the liver, the lymph nodes are grayish-yellow in color. As in the spleen, phagocytosis of erythrocytes is seen regularly (Schuchman 2001).

Histological examinations of the eye describe lipid-storing retinal ganglion cells as well as vacuolated cells in the different sections of the inner and outer layers of the ocular fundus. Lamellar deposits in cornea and lens epithelium can also be found histologically. Characteristic ocular changes have been demonstrated in a fetus as early as 23 weeks of gestation. By fundoscopy in patients with Niemann-Pick type A disease, the macular changes appear cherry-red as in Tay-Sachs disease. Visual acuity does not appear impaired. In contrast, in some patients who are not affected by the classic type A course, a halo-like grayish border is found around a less distinct intense red macular change. Some authors use the term *macula halo syndrome.* In addition, perifoveal punctate deposits are described by some authors in these patients. No systematic studies are available on the frequency of the ocular fundus changes in relation to the clinical presentation, especially neurological involvement. Thus, they are purely speculative. Clearly patients not affected by the classic type A course of Niemann-Pick disease also frequently show typical ocular fundus changes (Hammersen et al. 1979).

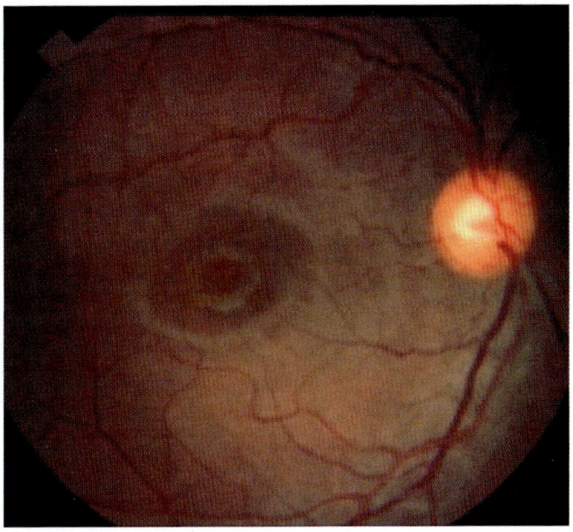

Figure 5.4: Ocular fundus with a so-called macula halo syndrome in a patient with intermediate course Niemann-Pick type A and B disease.

Most other organs also show the same histological changes to a lesser extent. However, their function is usually normal, e.g. kidney, pancreas, thyroid gland, etc. With thorough sample preparation, foam cells can also be found in the heart (Schuchman 2001).

Patients with intermediate, chronic neurological involvement have been reported only in individual case descriptions (Elleder et al. 1986, Ferlinz et al. 1995, Sogawa et al. 1978). Prospective, systematic studies in larger groups of patients have only been performed to describe visceral involvement (Wasserstein et al. 2003). Otherwise, numerous case reports (Candoni et al. 2001, Obenberger et al. 1999, Volders et al. 2002) and genetically oriented publications with retrospective, non-systematically collected, clinical data are available (Sikora et al. 2003, Simonaro et al. 2002). Apparently, neurological involvement does not directly correlate with visceral involvement. Some patients with intermediate course have significantly less visceral changes than patients with classic Niemann-Pick type B disease. Also, spleen and liver size as well as elevation of chitotriosidase activity and serum concentration do not differ. This leads to the assumption that different pathomechanisms control the expression of CNS involvement and visceral involvement.

Visceral involvement in patients with intermediate chronic neuropathic involvement is initially very pronounced and leads to diagnosis as early as infancy or preschool age. However, unlike patients with Niemann-Pick type B disease, in some cases the course is not continuously progressive. Some patients even showed decreasing spleen size in the second decade of life (Harzer et al. 2003). It is regularly noticed that the facial features are coarsened. Comparable characteristic changes are observed in Fabry disease.

These unusual courses are difficult to explain. Possibly, the imbalance between residual enzyme activity and visceral substrate formation (increased, age-dependent sphingomyelin turnover) is greater in these patients during infancy and preschool than during school age and adolescence. Strikingly, a so-called macula halo syndrome can be found very frequently in patients with an intermediate phenotype. This describes a gray shimmering ring in the form of a halo as retinal infiltration (☞ Figure 5.4).

An overview of the spectrum of **sphingomylinase deficiency** is provided by the following classification, which is adapted from Harzer et al. 2004. It differs from the description of the subtype categorization of McGovern and colleagues in that the chronic neurovisceral form of progression is divided into a significantly progressive and a mildly progressive form of course of the disease:

SMD 1

Acute, infantile, neuropathic sphingomyelinosis. Leading findings are failure to thrive, muscular hypotonia and development of severe global neurodegeneration. A cherry red spot (reddening of the fovea centralis) is frequently observed. Visceral involvement of the lungs, liver and spleen is very marked. Patients die in the first three years of life. The course is similar to Niemann-Pick type A disease.

SMD 2

Subacute, late infantile neuropathic sphingomyelinosis. Moderate to severe mental retardation, spastic cerebral palsy, vertical gaze palsy, macular halo syndrome and peripheral neuropathy are the neurologic findings. Visceral involvement is evident but not progressive, especially in the second decade of life. The course or progression is much slower than in SMD 1.

SMD 3

Chronic, neuropathic sphingomyelinosis. Mild mental retardation with slow progression and macula halo syndrome are the leading findings. Signs of peripheral neuropathy may be found but do not define the clinical picture. Mortality is mainly caused by visceral involvement.

SMD 4

Non-neuropathic form of progression. In the course, no or only very slight neurological symptoms (e.g., language development disorder, concentration deficits) are observed. Visceral involvement determines the clinical course. Survival is possible in individual cases until the fifth or sixth decade of life.

References

Candoni A, Grimaz S, Doretto P, Fanin R, Falcomer F, Bembi B. 2001. Sea-blue histiocytosis secondary to Niemann-Pick disease type B: a case report. Ann Hematol 80: 620-2

Elleder M, Nevoral J, Spicakova V, Hyniova H, Kraus J, et al. 1986. A new variant of sphingomyelinase deficiency (Niemann-Pick): visceromegaly, minimal neurological lesions and low in vivo degradation rate of sphingomyelin. J Inherit Metab Dis 9: 357-66

Ferlinz K, Hurwitz R, Weiler M, Suzuki K, Sandhoff K, Vanier MT. 1995. Molecular analysis of the acid sphingomyelinase deficiency in a family with an intermediate form of Niemann-Pick disease. Am J Hum Genet 56: 1343-9

Hammersen G, Oppermann HC, Harms E, Blassmann K, Harzer K. 1979. Oculo-neural involvement in an enzymatically proven case of Niemann-Pick disease type B. Eur J Pediatr 132: 77-84

Harzer K, Rolfs A, Bauer P, Zschiesche M, Mengel E, et al. 2003. Niemann-Pick disease type A and B are clinically but also enzymatically heterogeneous: pitfall in the laboratory diagnosis of sphingomyelinase deficiency associated with the mutation Q292 K. Neuropediatrics 34: 301-6

McGovern MM, et al. 2017. Consensus recommendation for a diagnostic guideline for acid sphingomyelinase deficiency. Genet Med 19(9): 967-74

Minai OA, Sullivan EJ, Stoller JK. 2000. Pulmonary involvement in Niemann-Pick disease: case report and literature review. Respir Med 94: 1241-51

Obenberger J, Seidl Z, Pavlu H, Elleder M. 1999. MRI in an unusually protracted neuronopathic variant of acid sphingomyelinase deficiency. Neuroradiology 41: 182-4

Schuchman EH, Desnick, R. J. 2001. Niemann-Pick disease types A and B: acid sphingomyelinase deficiencies. In:Scriver CR, Beaudet AL, Valle D, Sly WS (eds) The metabolic and molecular bases of inherited disease. McGraw Hill, New York.

Sikora J, Pavlu-Pereira H, Elleder M, Roelofs H, Wevers RA. 2003. Seven novel acid sphingomyelinase gene mutations in Niemann-Pick type A and B patients. Ann Hum Genet 67: 63-70

Simonaro CM, Desnick RJ, McGovern MM, Wasserstein MP, Schuchman EH. 2002. The demographics and distribution of type B Niemann-Pick disease: novel mutations lead to new genotype/phenotype correlations. Am J Hum Genet 71: 1413-9

Sogawa H, Horino K, Nakamura F, Kudoh T, Oyanagi K, et al. 1978. Chronic Niemann-Pick disease with sphingomyelinase deficiency in two brothers with mental retardation. Eur J Pediatr 128: 235-40

Takahashi T, Akiyama K, Tomihara M, Tokudome T, Nishinomiya F, et al. 1997. Heterogeneity of liver disorder in type B Niemann-Pick disease. Hum Pathol 28: 385-8

Volders P, Van Hove J, Lories RJ, Vandekerckhove P, Matthijs G, et al. 2002. Niemann-Pick disease type B: an unusual clinical presentation with multiple vertebral fractures. Am J Med Genet 109: 42-51

Wasserstein MP, Larkin AE, Glass RB, Schuchman EH, Desnick RJ, McGovern MM. 2003. Growth restriction in children with type B Niemann-Pick disease. J Pediatr 142: 424-8

5.2. Niemann-Pick type C disease

The clinical heterogeneity and variability concerning organ involvement, neurological symptoms and rate of progression is even more pronounced in Niemann-Pick type C disease than in type A + B disease. Both perinatal and manifestations over the age of 60 years are regularly observed in Niemann-Pick type C disease. The occurrence of visceral symptoms such as splenomegaly, prolonged jaundice and cholestatic hepatopathy does not indicate the neurological course that determines the disease. Only the age of manifestation and the phenotypic nature of the first neurological symptoms characterize the course of the disease.

The fact that the character of NPC changes from liver disease to neurodegenerative disease gave rise to the association with the chameleon. The chameleon changes color and is difficult to be found in its natural environment, thus symbolizing NPC.

Knowing well that the transitions are not always clearly delineated, a distinction into subgroups according to the age of manifestation of first neurological symptoms makes sense. This subclassification contains important information about morbidity and mortality and, in perspective, also about treatment options (Vanier and Millat 2003; ☞ Table 5.1).

5.2.1. Perinatal type

The perinatal manifestation corresponds to the nonspecific manifestation of severe infantile liver disease. With the improvement of diagnostic power and the increasingly widespread use of fetal ultrasonography examination, ascites is more frequently detected in utero in severely affected NPC patients. Prolonged jaundice with transition to cholestatic hepatopathy determines the course of

Age of onset	Neurological	Visceral	Course
Perinatal	• microcephaly (50 %) • problems with feeding • muscular hypotonia	• persistent fetal ascites • marked hepatosplenomegaly • prolonged jaundice • cholestatic hepatopathy, 20% liver failure • cystic lung lesion	• 20% die due to liver failure after 5 to 9 months • death due to pulmonary failure in case of lung involvement • neurologically corresponding manifestation in infancy (☞ below)
Infancy *Infantile onset*	• delayed motor development • hypotonia • ataxia	• hepatosplenomegaly	• transition to global encephalopathy • bulbar symptoms and pyramidal tract damage dominate the course of the disease • life expectancy 5-7 years
Early childhood *Late-infantile onset*	• cerebellar coordination disorder • slurred speech	• isolated splenomegaly • occasional hepatosplenomegaly • history of prolonged jaundice and/or passive cholestatic hepatopathy	• vertical supranuclear gaze palsy (VSGP) at approximately 6 years of age • transition to global encephalopathy • seizures accelerate the neurodegenerative course • bulbar symptoms and pyramidal tract damage dominate the course of the disease • life expectancy 10-15 years
School age *Juvenile onset*	• school failure • behavioral problems • VSGP • ataxia, dysarthria • dystonia • gelastic cataplexy • psychiatric symptoms	• mild splenomegaly • medical history of splenomegaly, prolonged jaundice or passive cholestatic hepatopathy	• transition to global encephalopathy • seizures accelerate neurodegenerative progression • dementia, bulbar symptoms and pyramidal tract damage dominate course • life expectancy 18-30 years
Adolescence and adulthood *Adult onset*	• psychosis • dementia • progressive cerebellar signs • progressive extrapyramidal and pyramidal signs		• transition to global encephalopathy • dementia, bulbar symptoms and pyramidal tract damage dominate the final stage • life expectancy 10-20 years after neurological manifestation

Table 5.1: Classification of Niemann-Pick type C disease according to manifestation of first neurological symptoms.

the disease in the first weeks of life and reflects severe liver involvement. For this reason, NPC disease must be included in the differential diagnosis of cholestatic hepatopathy in infancy (☞ Table 5.2). Muscular hypotonia with poor motor development in the first months of life must be considered a neurologic sign, although failure to thrive due to severe liver disease may influence this (Vanier and Millat 2003). Microcephaly is observed in approximately half of the cases.

Liver failure develops in approximately 20% of cases. Cases are repeatedly reported in which the diagnosis of NPC is made only after liver transplantation. But liver transplantation is not curative in NPC1 disease because the large membrane protein NPC1 cannot be integrated into host cells. Restorage in the donor liver occurs alongside unchanged neuropathic disease progression. In NPC2, curative therapy with hematologic stem cell transplantation is conceivable and has been performed in some individual cases.

Occasionally, pulmonary involvement is also observed in the perinatal manifestation. In specialised literature, NPC2 disease is almost exclusively reported in these cases. However, foam cell infiltration of the lung with radiologically palpable interstitial lung changes is also found in NPC1, but the changes in the lung scaffold are generally not as cystic and sometimes honeycombed as in NPC2. Lung involvement in NPC2 can lead to terminal lung failure (Bjurulf et al. 2008).

5.2.2. Infantile type

Pronounced hepatosplenomegaly is the leading finding in the infantile course type and usually prompts the pediatrician to take diagnostic steps in the first year of the patient's life. Usually, after exclusion of Gaucher and Niemann-Pick type A + B disease, diagnosis for NPC is initiated. Neurologic symptoms become evident by the end of the first year of life. Problems with sitting up and delayed achievement of motor milestones must be neuropediatrically interpreted as muscular hypotonia and motor developmental delay. Hearing loss is also frequently found on close examination. In contrast to later forms of progression, MRI imaging shows leukodystrophy, sometimes with cerebellar hypoplasia. In the further clinical course, there is initially a loss of acquired abilities (e.g., free standing). Cerebellar signs such as intention tremor and dysarthria are observed before pyramidal tract signs with marked spasticity dominate the course of the disease in the final stage. Bulbar signs, especially dysphagia with recurrent aspiration, aggravate the course and make normal oral feeding impossible. Usually, PEG placement with gastroesophageal reflux protection becomes necessary. Children die at preschool age (Iturriaga et al. 2006).

5.2.3. Late-infantile type

In most cases, splenomegaly precedes neurologic manifestation by 1-3 years. Normally, prolonged jaundice in the medical history is confirmed. At the onset of neurologic manifestation, parents report stumbling, clumsiness and gait unsteadiness at 3-5 years of age. A neuropediatric examination regularly diagnoses ataxia. Muscle tone may be decreased, so that joint malpositions with axial deviations – especially genu valgum ("knock-knees") and pes valgus ("flat feet") – lead to referral to an orthopedist. The vertical supranuclear gaze palsy (VSGP), typical for Niemann-Pick type C disease, is usually clearly noticeable at about 6 years of age. By accurate neuroophthalmologic examination, slowed and shortened saccades can be detected vertically but also horizontally 1-2 years before the manifestation of vertical gaze palsy.

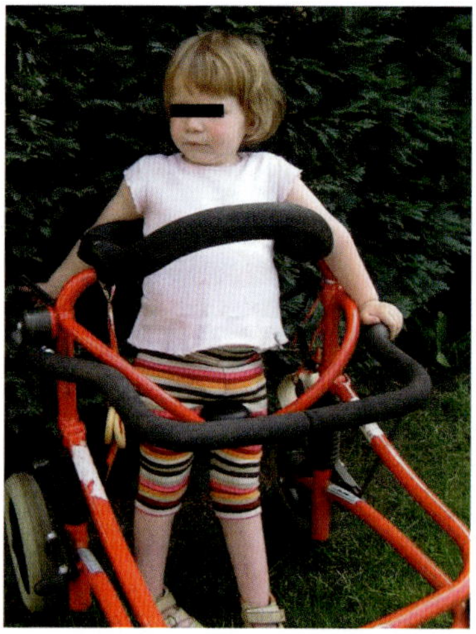

Figure 5.5: 4-year-old girl with late-infantile course. Clinically central hypotonia and ataxia. Walking is possible with an assistive device.

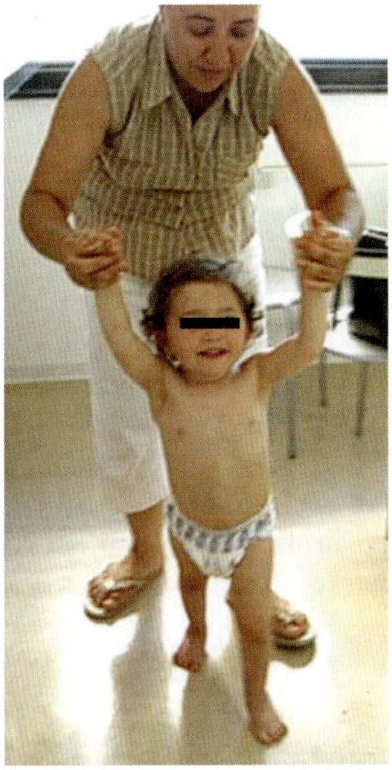

Figure 5.6a: 2-year-old girl with leading finding of muscular hypotonia in NPC. No independent free walking.

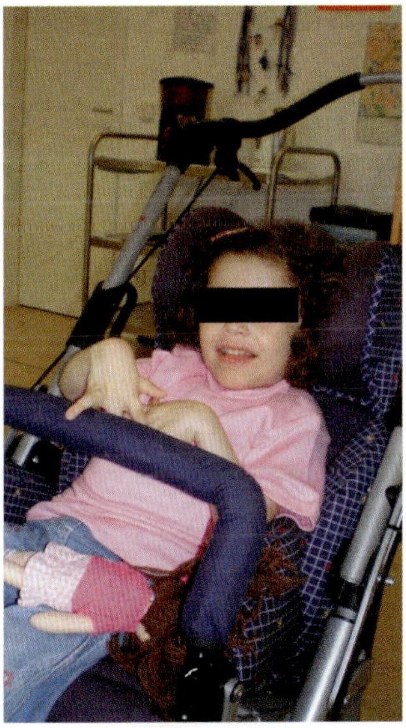

Figure 5.6b: Same child at age of 4 years. Now significant signs of spasticity and dystonic movement disorder.

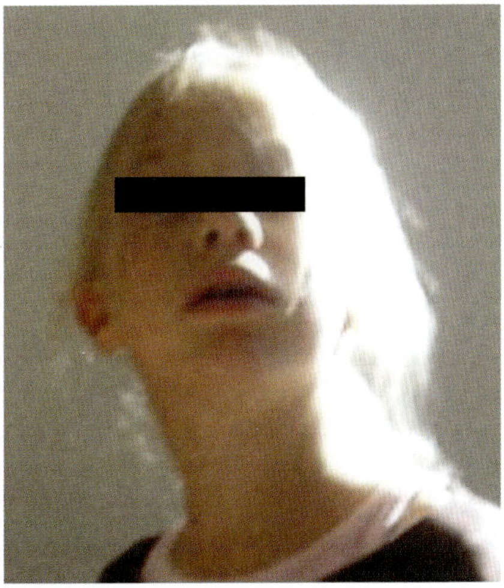

Figure 5.7: Female patient with juvenile course of Niemann-Pick type C with so-called underlooking, indicating vertical gaze paresis.

MRI imaging shows signal enhancement of the white matter in the T2-weighted image as seen in leukodystrophy.

Another typical neurological finding is gelastic cataplexy. In gelastic cataplexy, strong emotions, especially laughter, trigger sudden loss of tone while maintaining consciousness. To some extent, cataplexies are perceived as pleasant by the children and they learn to provoke them by stimulating laughter. The severity of the loss of tone can vary considerably. Often only head nodding is observed, but sometimes a complete falling seizure occurs, which carries a considerable risk of injury.

Cataplexy is defined according to the 3rd edition of the International Classification of Sleep Disorders (ICSD-3) as more than one episode of generally brief (<2 min), usually bilateral symmetrical sudden loss of muscle tone with preserved consciousness (Imanishi et al. 2020). The episodes are triggered by strong, often positive emotions, with almost all patients reporting that some episodes are triggered by laughter. The finding of a transient reversible loss of deep tendon reflexes during an episode, when observed, is a clear diagnostic clue. In children, cataplexy may present as facial (or generalized) hypotonia with drooping eyelids, open mouth and tongue hanging out, or gait unsteadiness shortly before the onset of disease. In children, anticipation of a reward is a common trigger. It is important to use child-appropriate context and language when attempting to obtain a history of cataplexy. Cataplexy is a prominent symptom that suggests narcolepsy cataplexy (= narcolepsy type 1, NT1). Cataplexy occurs in 26% of all NPC patients and is more common in patients with late-infantile onset (50%) and juvenile onset (38%) compared with patients with early-infantile onset (18%) and juvenile/adult onset (5%).

The pathophysiology of NPC is thought to lead to decreased orexin by damaging orexin-forming neurons. Orexin is a hypothalamic neuropeptide that specifically controls sleep-wake rhythm and muscle tone. Imanishi and coworkers found decreased orexin cerebrospinal fluid concentrations in NPC children with cataplexy (Imanishi et al. 2020).

In primary school age, partial and/or generalized seizures occur in more than 50% of children with preschool manifestations. Myoclonus is also regularly observed, but true myoclonus epilepsy is rare. As with other symptomatic epilepsies, a generalized seizure often occurs as the initial manifestation in the setting of a febrile infection or after sleep deprivation. Sometimes anticonvulsant treatment proves difficult. The EEG shows complex-focal changes.

The onset of epileptic seizures may be associated with rapid neurologic deterioration. Within a few months, marked cognitive deficits may develop,

Disease	Diagnosis	Characteristic sign	Treatment
Intrahepatic bile duct hypoplasia	histology after liver puncture	malabsorption	liver transplantation
Extrahepatic bile duct atresia	histology after liver puncture	malabsorption	liver transplantation
Type 1 tyrosinemia	amino acid analysis, succinylacetone test	hemorrhage	nitisinone
Cystic fibrosis	sweat testing, genetic testing	failure to thrive, bronchopulmonary infections	supportive
Progressive familial intrahepatic cholestasis	histology after liver puncture, gamma-GT normal, bile acids elevated	severe malabsorption	supportive, liver transplantation
Peroxisomal diseases, e.g. Zellweger syndrome	elevation of very long chain fatty acids (VLCFA) in plasma, special peroxisomal biochemistry (special laboratory)	cystic changes of liver and kidney in ultrasound imaging, encephalopathy	
NPC	filipin test (special laboratory), genetics	foam cells in bone marrow, hepatosplenomegaly	*NPC1* gene, *NPC2* gene
Alpha-1 antitrypsin deficiency	alpha-1 antitrypsin <70 mg/dL, ZZ mutation, serum electrophoresis		
Alagille syndrome	Clinical-genetic constellation of findings	pulmonary stenosis, wedge vertebrae	
Citrin deficiency	increase of citrulline, tyrosine, threonine, arginine and methionine, *CTLN2* gene	transitional infantile cholestasis, East Asian origin	
Classic galactosemia	enzyme activity, galactose and galactose-1-phosphate increased	direct hyperbilirubinemia, hemorrhage and vomiting after breast milk feed	galactose free diet

Table 5.2: Differential diagnosis of cholestatic hepatopathy in infancy.

and cerebellar signs, dystonic movement disorders, pyramidal tract signs and bulbar signs may also progress rapidly. Affected children, as well as their parents and families, experience a dramatic disrupture after a relatively stable phase, resulting in loss of independence and communication skills within a short period of time (Iturriaga et al. 2006, Vanier 2010).

5.2.4. Juvenile classic type

In the classic school-age manifestation, at least one common NPC-1 mutation is usually found. Many cases have a history of isolated splenomegaly at preschool age. Prolonged jaundice or a passive infantile cholestatic hepatopathy can be found in as many as 50% of juvenile cases. In few cases, differential diagnosis of splenomegaly by bone marrow aspiration or chitotriosidase measurement diagnoses NPC at the stage when neurologic signs are not yet present. More commonly, however, the diagnosis is delayed by 5-10 years. This means years of uncertainty for affected individuals with misdiagnosis and poorly targeted treatment (Imrie et al. 2007).

Typically, the diagnosis is made after elementary school age with the presence of characteristic neurological findings. At primary school age, the neurological symptoms are usually still very uncharacteristic and the focus lies on learning disabilities (Yanjanin et al. 2010).

Cerebellar signs

Motor unsteadiness and poor coordination are initially misdiagnosed as clumsiness and only diagnosed as ataxia when the gait pattern becomes conspicuous or dysarthria appears as a second cerebellar sign. An intention tremor can be traced on physical examination as a further cerebellar sign.

In a review article, Anheim and colleagues described the autosomal recessive disorders that are associated with ataxia and therefore must be considered as a differential diagnosis. They distinguished the autosomal recessive disorders from acquired ataxia disorders (e.g., cerebellitis in viral disease) and the autosomal dominant spinocerebellar ataxias (SCA). Niemann-Pick type C disease was assigned to autosomal recessive ataxia disorders without peripheral neuropathy. An overview is given in Table 5.3.

Vertical supranuclear gaze palsy (VSGP)

Supranuclear gaze palsies are due to dysfunctions in structures superior to the eye muscle nuclei in the upper brainstem. As a result, dysfunctions of saccade initiation, saccade amplitude and saccade velocity occur. Saccades are very fast, involuntary eye movements that humans use to adjust fixation to a new object. When this function is disrupted, noticeable head movements occur to fixate an object. In horizontal saccade disorder, head whirling is observed in affected individuals, and a tic disorder is often hypothesized. In VSGB, the phenomenon of *underlooking* is observed. When looking upward, the head is somewhat tilted. The patient seems be looking under something. Disturbed saccade initiation or speed is first discovered during a detailed neuroopthalmological examination, for example at school entry. A full-blown gaze paresis with disturbance of the voluntary gaze sequence movements is present at the age of 12-14 years. In most cases, horizontal supranuclear gaze palsy is also present. However, the typical symptoms are not as prominent as in Gaucher disease type III. Since the progression of horizontal saccade disorders can be better monitored by measuring saccade velocity and amplitude than vertical disorders, the neurological progression of the disease can be better assessed by diagnosing horizontal saccade disorders (Abel et al. 2009).

Disease progression

As the disease progresses, the occurrence of gelastic cataplexies and/or complex focal epilepsies is associated with marked clinical deterioration, cognitive decline and loss of elementary functions. Gelastic cataplexies are less common in juvenile than in late infantile courses. Affected families are not the only ones to notice dramatic progression of the disease. Dysphagia as a sign of brainstem involvement and incipient spasticity as a manifestation of pyramidal tract damage may develop slowly over years. Sometimes, however, these disorders become manifest over a few weeks in cases of poorly controllable epilepsy.

Dementia, cerebral palsy and bulbar inability to swallow characterize the final stage. A wheelchair is needed for mobility. Nutrition must be provided via PEG (percutaneous endoscopic gastrostomy). Aptly, NPC is sometimes referred to as Alzheimer's disease of the young.

Disease	Age	Clinical picture	MRT	Laboratory markers	Gene and protein
Cerebellar ataxia without peripheral neuropathy					
ARCA 1	20-40 years	only ataxia	cerebellar atrophy	-	SYNE1 (spectrin repeat containing nuclear envelope protein 1)
ARCA 2	1-10 years	mental retardation, myoclonus epilepsy	cerebellar atrophy, stroke-like lesions	lactate, Q10	ADCK3 (aarF domain containing kinase 3)
NPC	1-60 years	vertical supranuclear gaze palsy, splenomegaly, dystonia, cognitive decline	variable cerebellar and cerebral atrophy	filipin test	NPC1, NPC2
Cerebellar ataxia without sensoric neuropathy					
Friedreich's ataxia	7-25 years	hollow foot, scoliosis, behavioral changes	no cerebellar atrophy, spinal atrophy	-	FXN, frataxin
Sensory axonal neuropathy with dysarthria and ophtalmoplegia	20-60 years	ophthalmoplegia, dysarthria, ptosis, myoclonus	variable, white matter changes	lactate	polymerase gamma mutator (POLG), polymerase gamma
Vitamin E deficiency	2. decade	retinitis pigmentosa, tremor	no cerebellar atrophy, spinal atrophy	vitamin E	TTPA, alpha-tocopherol transfer protein
Abetalipoproteinemia	birth	neonatal steatorrhea	-	triglycerides	MTP, microsomal triglyceride transfer protein
Cerebellar ataxia with sensorimotor axonal neuropathy					
Ataxia telangioectasia	<5 years	Teleangiectasias, eye movement disorder, extrapyramidal movement disorder, infections, malignant diseases	cerebral atrophy	AFP, immunoglobulin	ATM
Ataxia with oculomotor apraxia type 1	1-20 years	oculomotor apraxia, chorea, dystonia	cerebral atrophy	variable LDL albumin	APTX, aprataxin
Ataxia with oculomotor apraxia type 2	7-25 years		cerebral atrophy	AFP	SETX, senataxin

Table 5.3: Autosomal recessive disorders associated with ataxia and therefore considered as a differential diagnosis to Niemann-Pick type C disease.

Psychiatric symptoms

In a recent publication, Sabine Sandu and coworkers showed that diagnostic delays occur especially (sometimes more than 10 years) when initial psychiatric symptoms determine the phenotype. In case series, psychiatric symptoms and findings were found in 30-40% of all patients with juvenile progressive form. In elementary school-aged children, cognitive deficits and behavioral problems with impulse control disorders may be misdiagnosed as autism spectrum disorder and attention deficit with or without hyperactivity as attention deficit hyperactivity syndrome (Sandu et al. 2009).

In adolescence, psychotic symptoms are psychiatrically prevalent along with behavioral problems with disinhibited social engagement. Paranoia, auditory and visual hallucinations, and, less frequently than in adulthood, sexual disinhibition may define the psychiatric symptoms.

Some patients appear very depressed and show little mood variation. Nevertheless, manifest bipolar disorders in adolescence have not been described so far.

Imaging

In the early phase of the disease, magnetic resonance imaging (MRI) can at best show a mildly characteristic atrophy of the cerebrum or cerebellar vermis. Since cerebellar vermis atrophy also occurs in other lysosomal storage diseases, this can at least be considered an indication. Occasionally, thinning of the corpus callosum is seen, but this is also not very pathognomonic. More typically, although only in advanced disease, signal enhancement in the posterior medullary canal may unmask secondary demyelination. In short, MRI imaging is of little use in diagnosing NPC disease, but may document the progression of CNS pathology.

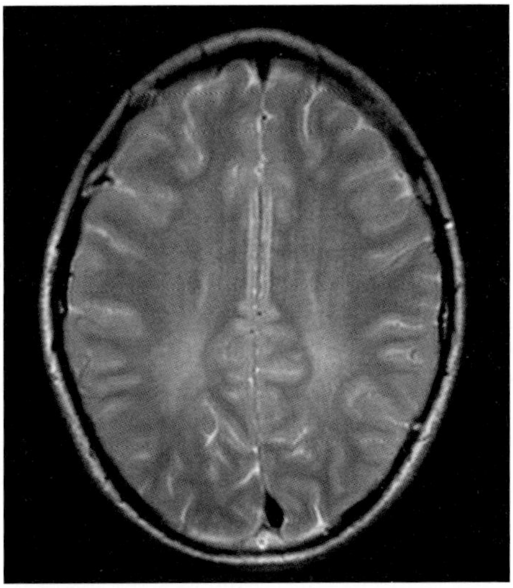

Figure 5.8: 15-year-old boy with juvenile course of Niemann-Pick type C disease. T2 weighted MRI coronary: hyperintense signal in white matter, occipital.

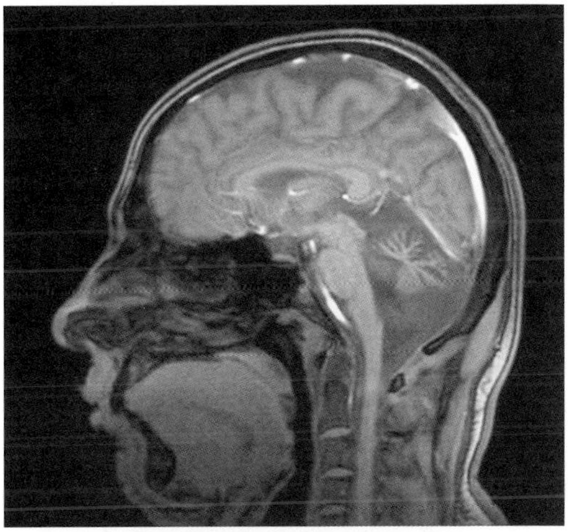

Figure 5.9: 17-year-old patient with juvenile course. Pronounced cerebellar atrophy. Marked ataxia for 5 years.

Proton magnetic resonance spectroscopy and diffusion tensor imaging (DTI) are newer investigative techniques that have been used in only a few studies in NPC. Initial results are promising. It may be possible to quantify pathologic changes with these techniques (Galanaud et al. 2009). However, their use in childhood and advanced disease is limited by the need for anesthesia to perform the examination. Anesthesia to perform diagnostics with no apparent benefit to the patient is an unacceptable risk.

5.2.5. Adult type

Although rare, inborn errors of metabolism are an important differential diagnosis in psychiatric and neuropsychiatric findings in adolescents and (young) adults. Niemann-Pick type C disease is an example of how inborn errors of metabolism can manifest with psychiatric or neuropsychiatric symptoms and findings at any age. Classic neurological findings, such as ataxia or dystonia, may not yet be pronounced, or may be mild, or may be misrecognized as drug side effects. In recent years, more and more adults are being diagnosed with subtle symptoms and findings. Both schizophrenic-psychotic and depressive pathologies are observed as initial symptoms of neurodegenerative disease. Ataxia and dystonia, as well as cognitive decline, may be superimposed on psychiatric symptoms or may develop later on. In addition, the rate of progression of neurological findings is much lower than in classic manifestations. Occasionally, visceral findings cannot be detected or are only apparent by sonography.

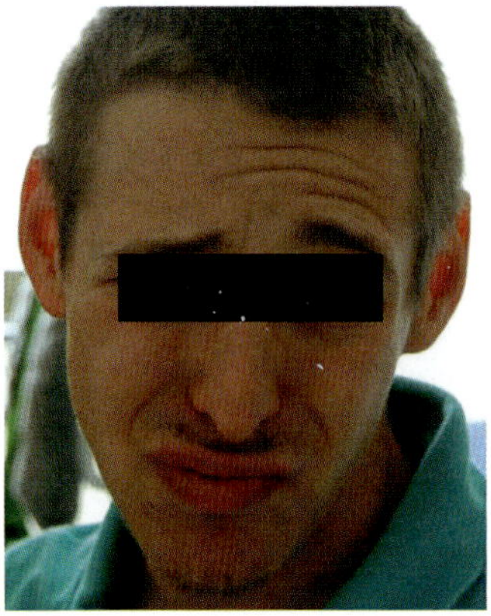

Figure 5.10: 17-year-old boy with facial dystonia in juvenile course of Niemann-Pick type C disease.

Mathieu Sevin and colleagues described a cohort of French adult NPC cases in Journal Brain in 2006. Evaluation figures are based on the 13 unrelated patients in the French cohort described in detail and an additional 55 cases published since 1969. The mean age (± standard deviation) at first neuropsychiatric symptoms is reported as 25 years (± 9.7 years). The delayed diagnosis, on average 6.2 years (± 6.4 years) later, highlights that this diagnosis is rarely thought of until characteristic symptoms are present, thus confirming the diagnosis is not straightforward.

The mean age at death of 38 years (± 10.2 years) is based on the analysis of only 20 cases. Due to this small number of cases, the survival time with the disease cannot be concluded (Sevin et al. 2007).

Major clinical findings are cerebellar ataxia (76%), vertical supranuclear gaze palsy (75%), movement disorders (58%), splenomegaly (54%), psychiatric disorders (45%) and dysphagia (37%). Epilepsy and cataplexy are rarely observed, in contrast to the juvenile manifestation. In their discussion, the authors distinguish between visceral findings and cortical and subcortical findings (☞ Table 5.4).

In the adult manifestation, visceral findings can be traced back to childhood in individual cases. Minor cortical signs in the sense of a learning disability are occasionally already apparent during school years. Subcortical findings dominate the progressive course of the disease in the later stages and are the cause of the lethal outcome. The variant biochemical phenotype appears to be less frequently associated with childhood splenomegaly and with fewer psychiatric symptoms. Mutations in the NPC-2 gene were found in only one of 33 cases.

In 2006, Mark Walterfang and colleagues reported on 3 young men who had been treated since adolescence for schizophrenia (2 patients) or bipolar disorder (1 patient). They developed neurological symptoms and cognitive deficits in early adult-

Visceral findings	Cortical findings	Subcortical findings
• splenomegaly • hepatomegaly	• psychiatric symptoms • cognitive deficits • epilepsy	• VSGP • cerebellar signs • movement disorders • dysphagia • cataplexy

Table 5.4: Differentiation between visceral, cortical and subcortical findings.

hood that eventually led to a diagnosis of NPC. Sexual disinhibition, auditory and visual hallucinations, persecutory delusions, catatonia, binge eating and manic episodes were found as psychiatric symptoms. Cognitive deficits were moderate to severe at the time of diagnosis. Dystonia, dysarthria, ataxia and VSNP were described as characteristic neurologic symptoms. The authors conclude that adolescents and young adults with chronic psychotic or affective disorders and cognitive deficits should be screened for NPC. A detailed neurological examination including neuro-ophthalmological testing is essential to establish the diagnosis.

References

Abel LA, Walterfang M, Fietz M, Bowman EA, Velakoulis D. 2009. Saccades in adult Niemann-Pick disease type C reflect frontal, brainstem, and biochemical deficits. Neurology 72: 1083-6

Bjurulf B, Spetalen S, Erichsen A, Vanier MT, Strom EH, Stromme P. 2008. Niemann-Pick disease type C2 presenting as fatal pulmonary alveolar lipoproteinosis: morphological findings in lung and nervous tissue. Med Sci Monit 14: CS71-5

Galanaud D, Tourbah A, Lehericy S, Leveque N, Heron B, et al. 2009. 24 month-treatment with miglustat of three patients with Niemann-Pick disease type C: follow up using brain spectroscopy. Mol Genet Metab 96: 55-8

Imanishi A, et al. 2020. Early detection of Niemann-pick disease type C with cataplexy and orexin levels: continuous observation with and without Miglustat. Orphanet J Rare Dis 15(1): 269

Imrie J, Dasgupta S, Besley GT, Harris C, Heptinstall L, et al. 2007. The natural history of Niemann-Pick disease type C in the UK. J Inherit Metab Dis 30: 51-9

Iturriaga C, Pineda M, Fernandez-Valero EM, Vanier MT, Coll MJ. 2006. Niemann-Pick C disease in Spain: clinical spectrum and development of a disability scale. Journal of the neurological sciences 249: 1-6

Sandu S, Jackowski-Dohrmann S, Ladner A, Haberhausen M, Bachmann C. 2009. Niemann-Pick disease type C1 presenting with psychosis in an adolescent male. Eur Child Adolesc Psychiatry 18: 583-5

Sevin M, Lesca G, Baumann N, Millat G, Lyon-Caen O, et al. 2007. The adult form of Niemann-Pick disease type C. Brain 130: 120-33

Vanier MT. 2010. Niemann-Pick disease type C. Orphanet J Rare Dis 5: 16

Vanier MT, Millat G. 2003. Niemann-Pick disease type C. Clin Genet 64: 269-81

Yanjanin NM, Velez JI, Gropman A, King K, Bianconi SE, et al. 2010. Linear clinical progression, independent of age of onset, in Niemann-Pick disease, type C. Am J Med Genet B Neuropsychiatr Genet 153B: 132-40

5.2.6. Psychiatric manifestations in Niemann-Pick type C disease

Psychiatric manifestations

At least one third of patients suffering from NPC show psychiatric symptoms many years before the onset of other features (Sevin et al. 2007, Vanier 2010). Such psychiatric signs manifest as psychoses such as paranoia, delusions, auditory and visual hallucinations, aggression and self-mutilation, and may also occur in combination with neurologically unremarkable manifestations (Josephs et al. 2003, Walterfang et al. 2006, Walterfang et al. 2010).

Further psychiatric manifestations include depressive syndromes and behavioral problems such as hypersexuality or social isolation. The onset of the disease in childhood is usually accompanied by mental as well as motor delay, gait and balance disturbances, seizures, ataxia, dystonia and vertical supranuclear gaze palsy. If the disease begins in adolescence or adulthood, symptoms manifest as neuropsychiatric disease or cognitive impairment (Patterson et al. 2004, Sevin et al. 2007, Vanier 2010, Walterfang et al. 2006). The neuropathological signs of NPC resemble a variety of other mental disorders. Many of the pathological changes that occur in the central nervous system (CNS) in these diseases are almost certainly responsible for the psychiatric manifestations of NPC. As a result of intracellular cholesterol blockade and impaired ability to transport endogenously synthesized cholesterol to distal axons, there is likely to be decreased supply to the membrane (Nixon 2004) and delayed response due to axonal impairment (Goodrum 1997). As a consequence of altered cholesterol levels, early axonal spheroid formation, hypomyelination or demyelination may be observed. Among these, axons and neurons in the corpus callosum, cerebellum, basal ganglia, and thalamus show the most striking axonal loss and frequently occur in NPC-related neuronal changes (German et al. 2002).

Magnetic resonance imaging (MRI) reveals a bilateral reduction of gray matter in functionally relevant brain regions of NPC patients. This reduction of gray matter in the hippocampus, thalamus, cerebellum and smaller regions of the inferoposterior cortex results in psychiatric and cognitive dysfunction (Walterfang et al. 2010).

Neurons affected due to NPC disease often show atrophied dendrites and significantly reduced dendritic arborization as a result of phosphorylation of microtubule-linked proteins (Fan et al. 2002, Walkley et al. 2004). These effects are similar to the structural changes seen in schizophrenia patients, which may also explain the neuropsychiatric symptoms (Kalus et al. 2000, Rosoklija et al. 2000).

Cholesterol is a major component of all cell membranes. Its accumulation is carefully regulated by the organism (Morell et al. 1996). The demand for cholesterol is particularly high during development in the central nervous system (CNS). The membrane of myelinated axons is dependent on endogenous cholesterol (Morell et al. 1996). Disturbances in cholesterol distribution and altered myelin content increase susceptibility to axonal impairment, which in turn is also a major feature of schizophrenia (Berger et al. 2002, Tkachev et al. 2003).

In mutations of the *NPC1* and *NPC2* genes, the onset of the disease usually manifests in adolescence or early adulthood. This is thought to be a consequence of impairment of the neuronal developmental process. This often results in altered myelination, impaired frontotemporal connectivity and impaired connectivity in the striatum, which in turn may cause neuropsychiatric symptoms in the patient (Berger et al. 2002, Benes 1989, Friston et al. 1995, Pantelis et al. 1997). Compared to other genetic disorders affecting the white matter and metachromatic leukodystrophies, neuropsychiatric symptoms are equally common in Niemann-Pick type C.

Accumulation of cholesterol, glycolipids and GM_2 or GM_3 gangliosides in late endosomes leads to neurofibrillary changes, neuronal degeneration and demyelination, similar to Alzheimer's disease (Nixon 2004, Pacheco et al. 2009). However, these symptoms may be worsened by involvement of apolipoprotein E (*ApoE4*), which is important for metabolism and lipoprotein transport.

Recent evidence suggests that *ApoE4* has an accelerating effect with respect to the accumulation of amyloid-beta-42 peptides in early endosomes. One possible consequence is presenilin-1 redistribution to early endosomes in NPC patients and an increase in gamma-secretase activity (Burns et al. 2003, Kuo et al. 1998). Homozygous *ApoE4* alleles lead to amyloid-beta deposition and accelerate the accumulation of abnormally phosphorilated tau in neurons in patients with mutations in the *NPC1* gene (Saito et al. 2002).

Neuropsychiatric manifestations in NPC-affected individuals arise due to dysfunctional axonal structures that spread to cortical and subcortical structures in the presence of total axonal loss as well as specific neurodegeneration.

NPC clinically presents in a very heterogeneous manner. The age at which the disease presents ranges from the perinatal period to adulthood. The onset of symptoms may also differ by years in siblings. In addition, considerable phenotypic variability is seen in siblings.

Almost all NPC patients develop neurologic and/or psychiatric symptoms. Psychiatric manifestations can therefore occur in NPC patients both at the onset of adulthood and as early as adolescence. In the current literature, neuropsychiatric symptoms such as auditory hallucinations, paranoid delusions, and formal and content thinking disorders (Josephs et al. 2003, Sandu et al. 2009, Sevin et al. 2007) have been observed in more than 30 cases before and after confirmed NPC diagnosis (☞ Table 5.5).

These psychiatric manifestations may persist on their own for many years and/or be associated with psychotic symptoms (paranoid delusions, auditory or visual hallucinations, non-hallucinatory thought disorder, behavioral disturbances such as aggression, self-mutilation or social isolation) before being associated with NPC disorder.

People with onset of the disease in adulthood are therefore difficult to diagnose, especially if they have psychotic disorders. In the past, these patients were prescribed neuroleptics, which in turn led to the development of dyskinesia.

For this reason, it is very important to be vigilant for psychotic manifestations in NPC patients, as they may be particularly prominent, especially in the adult form. An earlier case report by Shulman and colleagues (1995) described a 38-year-old Peruvian man who had to live with the misdiagnosis of chronic schizophrenia for eight years because of initial signs of psychosis. This case alone calls for clarification and for a search for more details in cases of NPC with disease onset in adulthood. From these retrospective case reports in the medical literature, six additional individuals with psychiatric signs were identified. Of these six cases, four initially received a diagnosis of psychosis before then being correctly diagnosed with NPC disease. At that time, there was an average delay of 6 to 12 years between initial onset of signs and diagnosis (Vanier et al. 1991, Vanier et al. 1988, Yan-Go et al. 1984).

Based on further studies in the following years, young adults were identified who initially showed neuropsychiatric symptoms such as paranoid schizophrenia, auditory and visual hallucinations.

Case	Gender	Age of onset (years	Age of diagnosis (years)	Psychiatric manifestation (before NPC diagnosis)	Psychiatric manifestation (after NPC diagnosis)	References
1	M	13	13		X	Walterfang, 2010
2	M	7	17	X		Sandu, 2009
3	M	16	25	X		Sevin, 2007
4	F	30	40	X		Sevin, 2007
5	M	12	15		X	Sevin, 2007
6	F	16	29	X		Sevin, 2007
7	M	3			X	Sevin, 2007
8	M		10		X	Sevin, 2007
9	M	16	24	X		Walterfang, 2006
10	M	15	23		X	Walterfang, 2006
11	M				X	Walterfang, 2006
12	F	53	68	X		Trendelenburg, 2006
13	M	23		X		Sullivan, 2005
14	M	25	33	X		Battisti, 2003
15	F	49	61	X		Josephs, 2003
16	F	27	32	X		Josephs, 2003
17	F	20	23	X		Imrie, 2002
18	M	21	22	X		Imrie, 2002
19	F	7			X	Imrie, 2002
20	M	14			X	Imrie, 2002
21	M	17	0	X		Imrie, 2002
22	F	18	25	X		Imrie, 2002
23	M	16	0	X		Campo, 1998
24	M	17	22	X		Love, 1995
25	M	18	20	X		Love, 1995
26	M	30	38		X	Shulman, 1995
27	M	19	32	X		Vanier, 1991
28	M	45		X		Vanier, 1991
29	F	34		X		Vanier, 1991
30	NA	28			X	Vanier, 1988
31	F	18	21		X	Yan-Go, 1984
32	F	40	41	X	X	Klünemann, 2002
33	F	35	43	X	X	Klünemann, 2002

Table 5.5: Case reports of psychiatric manifestations in the past 25 years, before and after Niemann-Pick diagnosis with disease onset in adolescence or adulthood.

The time between the onset of psychiatric symptoms and confirmation of an NPC disorder has been estimated to range from 4 to 10 years (Walterfang et al. 2006, Campo et al. 1998, Sandu et al. 2009).

These cases highlight the importance of veryfing diagnoses of patients with combinations of psychoses, cognitive and motor disorders. Because of this, a particularly precise approach to psychiatric diagnosis is essential when patients also present with discrete neurological symptoms.

A number of studies have looked at different populations and found that approximately 40% of NPC patients whose onset was in adolescence or adulthood and whose initial symptoms resembled psychosis did not have neurologically abnormal examination scores. Therefore, the diagnoses for these patients were schizophrenia or another psychotic subcategory. A recently published study of 13 French NPC patients in adolescence and adulthood identified six affected individuals with abnormal psychiatric or cognitive symptoms (Sevin et al. 2007). The study further reported two patients with psychiatric symptoms, including paranoid schizophrenia. They could only be diagnosed with NPC retrospectively (Sevin et al. 2007). Another study examined individuals with NPC between 1976 and 2000 at the Mayo Clinic in Rochester, USA (Josephs et al. 2003). The investigators were able to locate five individuals whose onset of disease was in adulthood and two of whom were initially diagnosed with psychosis. One person was a 32-year-old woman who had been diagnosed with a neuropsychiatric disorder and was only told of the actual diagnosis of NPC five years later.

The second person was a 61-year-old woman who lived without a clear diagnosis for 15 years, only aware of a progressive neuropsychiatric disorder, before she was also diagnosed with NPC (Josephs et al. 2003).

These examples illustrate both the wide age range of NPC and the time that can lapse before affected individuals receive a clear diagnosis (Josephs et al. 2003).

Imrie and colleagues (2002) confirmed the early finding that psychiatric manifestations are a common presentation in NPC patients with disease onset in adolescence and adulthood.

As result of the examination of 17 cases of people with NPC, seven individuals were identified in whom neuropsychotic symptoms were clearly evident at isolated points in the disease. Four individuals presented psychoses with visual hallucinations and delusions, which also preceded a diagnosis of NPC in this case (Imrie et al. 2002). Psychosis tends to occur later in the presentation of an NPC patient when onset occurs in adolescence or adulthood.

The intake of neuroleptics leads to an improvement of psychiatric symptoms (Sandu et al. 2009, Josephs et al. 2003).

A study by Walterfang et al. (2010) reported on a pubescent boy with disease onset in adolescence. The patient developed seizure-like psychiatric symptoms including visual and auditory hallucinations. His psychoses were treated long-term with valproate. However, confusion was always present postictally (Walterfang et al. 2010).

In general, NPC as well as related storage disorders must be considered when diagnosing psychosis in adolescents. This is especially true when psychosis develops in association with movement disorders or there is evidence of cognitive impairment. Despite its rarity, NPC should be ruled out by child and adolescent psychiatrists through case taking and neurologic testing. This could prevent initial misdiagnosis such as schizophrenia and avoid application of inappropriate medication to patients.

Current treatment options and management of the psychiatric components of the disease

Only recently, new therapies have been developed that have already delayed the progression of the disease in animal studies (Ahmad et al. 2005, Bascunan-Castillo et al. 2004). Although research continues to improve medications, important information regarding neuropsychological testing parameters for people with NPC is still lacking. For clinical investigations of new treatments, diagnostically appropriate techniques are needed that are based on neuropsychological parameters and therefore produce reliable measurement results. A study published in 2007 attempted to address this issue by compiling a neuropsychological test battery. The aim was to determine whether specific deficits could be associated with individual stages

Early stage Few behavioral changes are noticed in the individual:
Verbal Fluency, Trail Making Test A & B, Grooved Pegboard, memory (e.g. CERAD word list memory, recall, recognition)
Intermediate stage Significant behavioral abnormalities occur in the individual:
MMST, Constructional Praxis, Grooved Pegboard, Boston Naming, Trail Making Test A&B, memory (e.g. CERAD word list memory, recall, recognition)
Late stage The individual is extremely limited in his behavior and abilities:
MMST, Corsi Block-Tapping Test, Trail Making Test A & B, Constructional Praxis, Boston Naming or *MMST, Severe Impairment Battery, Peabody Picture Vocabulary Test, Constructional Practise*

Table 5.6: Neuropsychological testing procedures for the diagnosis of NPC disorder.

of the disease (Hinton et al. 2005; Klarner et al. 2007).

Klarner et al. (2007) concluded that there was no neuropsychological test that could be used with all stages of NPC. *Trail Making Test A and B* and *Verbal fluency* were good indicators of the early stages of the disease, while the *CORSI Blocktapping, Mini Mental Status, Find Similarities,* and *Clock Drawing Test* showed abnormal results in advanced stages (Klarner et al. 2007). Cognitive tasks and fine motor skills were measured using the *Grooved Pegboard, Trail Making,* and the *Mosaic Test,* but turned out to be unsuitable because differences in cognitive and fine motor symptoms of the disease were difficult to interpret (Klarner et al. 2007). In general, however, further studies need to be conducted in this area to ultimately establish a valid and appropriate neuropsychological test battery for the examination of Niemann-Pick type C patients.

Thus, there are significant challenges for the clinical management of NPC patients, as the disease is very heterogeneous as well as relatively rare, the symptoms appear nonspecific, and it takes a long time to reach a diagnosis. In addition, there is currently a lack of therapeutic monitoring and control options.

In most countries, in addition to local care by specialists, treatment is also provided in specialized centers. However, support for these options is still hampered due to the lack of national and international guidelines to prescribe specific treatment for the disease. Pharmaceutical treatments have now been developed to treat the symptoms and various manifestations of NPC disease (Patterson et al. 2004, Wraith et al. 2009).

Cataplexy, the abrupt reversible loss of muscle tone while fully conscious, for example, is controlled by tricyclic antidepressants such as amytriptyline or clomipramine (Patterson et al. (eds.), Kandt et al. 1982).

However, as has recently been found, tricyclic antidepressants are probably not appropriate. The drug imipramine causes symptoms similar to NPC in cell culture. Antiepileptic drugs are commonly used to control or reduce the incidence of seizures, meanwhile insomnia is treated with melatonin. Symptoms such as dystonia and tremor appear in early stages of the disease and can be relieved with anticholinergics, beta-blockers and anticonvulsants. In some cases, dystonia can also be treated with levodopa (Josephs et al. 2003).

Physiotherapy can lead to a reduction in tremor and an improvement in coordination as well as muscle control. Speech therapy minimizes the risk of aspiration.

Neuropsychiatric schizophrenic manifestations that occur at onset in adolescence and adulthood can be treated like other antipsychotic diseases if no other manifestations are noted.

Thioridazine and haloperidol are often prescribed as antipsychotics. However, these may worsen tremors and dyskinesias (Josephs et al. 2003).

Valproate has been prescribed to reduce seizure-like psychotic symptoms (Walterfang et al. 2010).

Recent animal studies using NPC1 transgenic mice indicate that the reduced neuropsychiatric symptoms observed in patients are likely a result of improvement in neuronal differentiation, restoration of impaired astrocytes and reduction in cholesterol levels (Walterfang et al. 2010, Kim et al. 2007).

The most significant advance in the treatment of neurologic manifestations in adults and children with NPC has been the development of miglustat. Miglustat is used for substrate reduction therapy, as it is an iminosugar that acts as a reversible competitive inhibitor of glucosylkeramide synthesis.

This results in reduced production of neurotoxic GM_2 and GM_3 gangliosides (Butters et al. 2000, Platt et al. 1994a, Platt et al. 1994b). Miglustat is able to cross the blood-brain barriera, leading to a reduction in the accumulation of glycosphingolipids and pathological cell tissue. This in turn delays neurological symptoms and increases survival (Patterson et al. 2007, Patterson et al. 2010, Pineda et al. 2009, Wraith et al. 2010). Miglustat reduces the incidence of psychiatric symptoms and is also well tolerated by children and adolescents with NPC. Side effects may include gastrointestinal distress and tremor (Patterson et al. 2007, Pineda et al. 2009, Pineda et al. 2010).

References

Ahmad I, Lope-Piedrafita S, Bi X, et al. 2005. Allopregnanolone treatment, both as a single injection or repetitively, delays demyelination and enhances servival of Niemann-Pick C mice. J Neurosci Res 82: 811-21

Bascunan-Castillo EC, Erickson RP, Howison CM, et al. 2004. Tamoxifen and vitamin E treatments delay symptoms in the mouse model of Niemann-Pick C. J Appl Genet 45: 461-7

Benes FM. 1989. Myelination of cortical-hippocampal relays during late adolescence. Schizophr Bull 15: 585-93

Berger GE, Wood SJ, Pantelis C, et al. 2002. Implications of lipid biology for the pathogenesis of schizophrenia. Aust N Z J Psychiatry 36: 355-66

Burns M, Gaynor K, Olm V, et al. 2003. Presenilin redistribution associated with aberrant cholesterol transport enhances beta-amyloid production in vivo. J Neurosci 23: 5645-9

Butters TD, Dwek RA, Platt FM. 2000. Inhibition of glycosphingolipid biosynthesis: application to lysosomal storage disorders. Chem Rev 100: 4683-96

Campo JV, Stowe R, Slomka G, et al. 1998. Psychosis as a presentation pf physical disease in adolescence: a case of Niemann-Pick disease, type C. Dev Med Neurol 40: 126-9

Fan QW, YU W, Gong JS, et al. 2002. Cholesterol-dependent modulation of dendrite outgrowth and microtubule stability in cultured neurons. J Neurochem 80: 178-90

Friston KJ, Frith CD. 1995. Schizophrenia: a disconnection syndrome? Clin Neurosci 3: 89-97

German DC, Liang CL, Song T, et al. 2002. Neurodegenreation in the Niemann-Pick C mouse: glial involvement. Neuroscience 109: 437-50

Goodrum JF, Pentchev PG. 1997. Cholesterol reutilization during myelination of regenerating PNS axons is impaired in Niemann-Pick disease type C mice. J Neurosci Res. 49: 389-92

Hinton V, Vecchino D, Prady H, et al. 2005. The cognitive phenotype of type C disease: neuropsychological characteristics of patients at baseline in a clinical trial with oral miglustat. American Society of Human Genetics, Conference, Salt Lake City, Utah

Imanishi A, et al. 2020. Early detection of Niemann-pick disease type C with cataplexy and orexin levels: continuous observation with and without Miglustat. Orphanet J Rare Dis 15(1): 269

Imrie J, Vijayaraghaven S, Whitehouse C, et al. 2002. Niemann-Pick disease type C in adults. J Inherit Metab Dis 25: 491-500

Josephs KA, Van Gerpen MW, Van Gerpen JA. 2003. Adult onset Niemann-Pick disease type C presenting with psychosis. J Neurol Neurosurg Psychiatry 74: 528-9

Kalus P, Muller TJ, Zuschratter W, et al. 2000. The dendritic architecture of prefrontal pyramidal neurons in schizophrenic patients. Neuroreport 11: 3621-5

Kandt RS, Emerson RG, Singer HS, et al. 1982. Cataplexy in variant forms of Niemann-Pick disease. Ann Neurol 12: 284-8

Kim SJ, Lee BH, Lee YS, et al. 2007. Defective cholesterol traffic and neuronal differentiation in neural stern cells of Niemann-Pick type C disease improved by valproic acid, a histone deacetylase inhibitor. Biochem Biophys Res Commun 360: 593-9

Klarner B, Kluenemann HH, Lurding R, et al. 2007. Neuropsychological profile of adult patients with Niemann-Pick C1 (NPC1) mutations. J Inherit Metab Dis 30: 60-7

Kuo YM, Emmerling MR, Bisgaier CL, et al. 1998. Elevated lowdensity lipoprotein in Alzheimer´s disease correlates with brain abeta 1-42 levels. Biochem Biophys Res Commun 252: 711-5

McGovern MM, et al. 2017. Consensus recommendation for a diagnostic guideline for acid sphingomyelinase deficiency. Genet Med 19(9): 967-74

Mengel E, et al. 2013. Niemann-Pick disease type C symptomatology: an expert-based clinical description. Orphanet J Rare Dis 8: 166

Morell P, Jurevics H. 1996. Origin of cholesterol in myelin. Neurochem Res 21: 463-70

Nixon RA. 2004. Niemann-Pick type C disease and Alzheimer´s disease: the APP-endosome connection fattens up. Am J Pathol 164: 757-61

Pacheco CD, Elrick MJ, Lieberman AP. 2009. Tau deletion exacerbates the phenotype of Niemann-Pick type C mice and implicates autophagy in pathogenesis. Hum Mol Genet 18: 956-65

Pantelis C, Barnes TR, Nelson HE, et al. 1997. Frontal-striatal cognitive deficits in patients with chronic schizophrenia. Brain 120(10): 1823-43

Patterson MC, Vanier MT, Suzuki K, et al. (eds). Niemann-Pick disease type C: a lipid trafficking disorder. The Metabolic and Molecular Bases of Inherited Disease, New York: McGraw Hill 16(145): 3611-33

Patterson MC, Platt F. 2004. Therapy of Niemann-Pick disease, type C. Biochim Biophys Acta 1685: 77-82

Patterson MC, Vecchio D, Prady H, et al. 2007. Miglustat for treatment of Niemann-Pick C disease: a randomised controller study. Lancet Neurol 6: 765-72

Patterson MC, Vecchio D, Jacklin E, et al. 2010. Long-term miglustat therapy in children with Niemann-Pick disease type C. J Child Neurol 25: 300-5

Pineda M, Wraith JE, Mengel E, et al. 2009. Miglustat in patients with Niemann-Pick disease Type C (NP-C): a multicenter observational retrospective cohort study. Mol Genet Metab 98: 243-9

Pineda M, Perez-Poyato MS, O´Callaghan M, et al. 2010. Clinical experience with miglustat therapy in pediatric patients with Niemann-Pick disease type C: a case series. Mol Genet Metab 99: 358-66

Platt FM, Neises GR, Dwek RA, et al. 1994a. N-butyldeoxynojirimycin is a novel inhibitor of glycolipid biosynthesis. J Biol Chem 269: 8362-5

Platt FM, Neises GR, Karlsson GB, et al. 1994b. N-butyldeoxygalactonojirimycin inhibits glycolipid biosynthesis but does not affect N-linked oligosaccharide processing. J Biol Chem 269: 27108-14

Rosoklija G, Toomayan G, Ellis SP, et al. 2000. Structural abnormalities of subicular dendrites in subjects with schizophrenia and mood disorders : Preliminary findings. Arch Gen Psychiatry 57: 349-56

Saito Y, Suzuki K, Nanba E, et al. 2002. Niemann-Pick type C disease : accelerated neurofibrillary tangle formation and amyloid beta deposition associated with apolipoprotein E epsilon 4 homozygosity. Ann Neurol 52: 351-5

Sandu S, Jackowski-Dohrmann S, Ladner A, et al. 2009. Niemann-Pick disease type C1 presenting with psychosis in an adolescent male. Eur Child Adolesc Psychiatry 18: 583-5

Sevin M, Lesca G, Baumann N, et al. 2007. The adult form of Niemann-Pick disease type C. Brain 130: 120-33

Shulman LM, David NJ, Weiner WJ. 1995. Psychosis as the initial manifestation of adult-onset Niemann-Pick disease type C. Neurology 45: 1739-43

Tkachev D, Mimmack ML, Ryan MM, et al. 2003. Oligodendrocyte dysfunction in schizophrenia and bipolar disorder. Lancet 362: 798-805

Vanier MT, Wenger DA, Comly ME, et al. 1988. Niemann-Pick disease group C: clinical variability and diagnosis based on defective cholesterol esterification. A collaborativestudy on 70 patients. Clin Genet 33: 331-48

Vanier MT, Rodriguez-Lafrasse C, Rousson R, et al. 1991. Type C Niemann-Pick disease : sprectrum of phenotypic variation in disruption of intracellular LDL-derived cholesterol processing. Biochim Biophys Acta, 1096: 328-37

Vanier MT. 2010. Niemann-Pick disease type C. Orphanet J Rare Dis 5: 16

Walkley SU, Suzuki K. 2004. Consequences of NPC1 and NPC2 loss of function in mammalian neurons. Biochim Biophys Acta 1685: 48-62

Walterfang M, Fietz M, Fahey M, et al. 2006. The neuropsychiatry of Niemann-Pick type C disease in adulthood. J Neuropsychiatry Clin Neurosci 18: 158-70

Walterfang M, Kornberg A, Adams S, et al. 2010. Postictal psychosis in adolescent Niemann-Pick disease type C. [Electronic version]. J Inherit Metab Dis

Wraith JE, Baumgartner MR, Bembi B, et al. 2009. Recommendations on the diagnosis and management of Niemann-Pick disease type C. Mol Genet Metab 98: 152-65

Wraith JE, Vecchio D, Jacklin E, et al. 2010. Miglustat in adult and juvenile patients with Niemann-Pick disease type C : long-term data from a clinical trial. Mol Genet Metab 99: 351-7

Yan-Go Fl, Yanagihara T, Pierre RV, et al. 1984. A progressive neurologic dosorder with supranuclear vertical gaze paresis and distinctive bone marrow cells. Mayo Clin Proc 59: 404-10

References for Table 5.5

Battisti C, Tarugi P, DottiMT, et al. 2003. Adult onset Niemann-Pick type C disease: A clinical neuroimaging and molecular genetic study. Mov Disord 18: 1405-9

Campo JV, Stowe R, Slornka G, et al. 1998. Psychosis as a presentation of physical disease in adolescence. A case of Niemann-Pick disease type C. Dev Med Child Neurol 40: 126-9

Imrie J, Vijayaraghaven S, Whitehouse C, et al. 2002. Niemann-Pick disease type C in adults. J Inherit Metab Dis 25: 491-500

Josephs KA, Van Gerpen MW, Van Gerpen JA. 2003. Adult onset Niemann-Pick disease type C presenting with psychosis. J Neurol Neurosurg Psychiatry 74: 528-9

Klünemann HH, Elleder M, Kaminski WE, Snow K, Peyser JM, O'Brien JF, Munoz D, Schmitz G, Klein HE & Pendlebury WW. 2002. Frontal lobe atrophy due to a mutation in the cholesterol binding protein HE1/NPC2. Ann Neurol 52: 743-749

Love S, Bridges LR, Case CP. 1995. Neurofibrillary tangles in Niemann-Pick disease type C. Brain 118(Pt1): 119-29

Sandu S, Jackowski-Dohrmann S, Ladner A, et al. 2009. Niemann-Pick disease type C1 presenting with psychosis in an adolescent male. Eur Child Adolesc Psychiatry 18: 583-5

Sevin M, Lesca G, Baumann N, et al. 2007. The adult form of Niemann-Pick disease type C. Brain 130: 120-33

Shulman LM, David NJ, Weiner WJ. 1995. Psychosis as the initial manifestation of adult-onset Niemann-Pick disease type C. Neurology 45: 1739-43

Sullivan D, Walterfang M, Velakoulis D. 2005. Bipolar disorders and Niemann-Pick disease type C. Am J Psychiatry 162: 1021-2

Trendelenburg G, Vanier MT, Maza S, et al. 2006. Niemann-Pick type C disease in a 68-year-old patient. J Neurol Neurosurg Psychiatry 77: 997-8

Vanier MT, Wenger DA, Comly ME, et al. 1988. Niemann-Pick disease group C: clinical variability and diagnosis based on defectivecholesterol esterification. A collaborative study on 70 patients. Clin Genet 33: 331-48

Vanier MT, Rodriguez-Lafrasse C, Rousson R, et al. 1991. Type C Niemann-Pick disease : biochemical aspects and phenotypic heterogeneity. Dev Neurosci 13: 307-14

Walterfang M, Fietz M, Fahey M, et al. 2006. The neuropsychiatry of Niemann-Pick type C disease in adulthood. J Neuropsychiatry Clin Neurosci 18: 158-70

Walterfang M, Kornberg A, Adams S et al. 2010. The neuropsychiatry of Niemann-Pick disease type C. J Inherit Metab Dis [Epub ahead of print]

Yan-Go FL, Yanagihara T, Pierre RV, et al. 1984. A progressive neurologic disorder with supranuclear vertical gaze paresis and distinctive bone marrow cells. Mavo Clin Proc 59: 404-10

Management and treatment of Niemann-Pick diseases

6. Management and treatment of Niemann-Pick diseases

6.1. Management and treatment of Niemann-Pick type A/B disease

No causative and effective treatment is available for Niemann-Pick type A and B disease (acid sphingomyelinase deficiency, ASMD). Management is aimed at symptomatic support and reduction of complications of the disease. This chapter provides some useful guidance on the care and supportive therapy of patients with the full spectrum of sphingomyelinase deficiency. The notes were developed in the long-term care of more than 40 patients over more than 20 years. Scientifically based recommendations for the care of ASMD patients were published in 2019 (Wasserstein et al. 2019).

The infantile, neurovisceral form of disease (type A) is comparatively uniform. The children mostly die by 3 years of age. Palliative challenges include failure to thrive, dyspnea, spasticity and dysphagia. In contrast, chronic neurovisceral and visceral progressions have significant disease-specific organ manifestations that require supportive care.

Monitoring strategies are presented in the following sections. Supportive treatments and/or lifestyle changes aim to alleviate the impact of symptoms.

6.1.1. Supportive care

Hepatic insufficiency

Hepatic and pulmonary insufficiency are the most common causes of death in patients with Niemann-Pick type B disease. Cassiman et al. examined the causes of death in ASMD in an international multicenter study. The overall leading causes of death were respiratory as well as liver failure (27.7% each), regardless of age. In patients with chronic neurovisceral ASMD, progression to neurodegenerative disease was a leading cause of death, along with respiratory disease (both 23.1%) and liver disease (19.2%). As with other liver diseases, alcohol abuse, medications and infections with hepatitis viruses can accelerate progression. A causal therapy is not yet available. Liver transplantation has not been proven to be effective. In most cases, the general condition at this stage of the disease is so poor, especially due to lung involvement, that liver transplantation is not feasible anyway.

Bronchoalveolar lavage

Temporary improvement of symptoms such as susceptibility to infection, cyanosis and dyspnea caused by lung infiltration of storage cells can be achieved by bronchiopulmonary lavage (Nicholson et al. 2002). Since the memory cells infiltrate the lungs again after months, the effect does not appear to be persistent (☞ Figure 6.1). The microscopic image shows storage cells in the lavage fluid. The child had 8 pneumonias requiring antibiotic treatment in the year before lavage and only one in the year after.

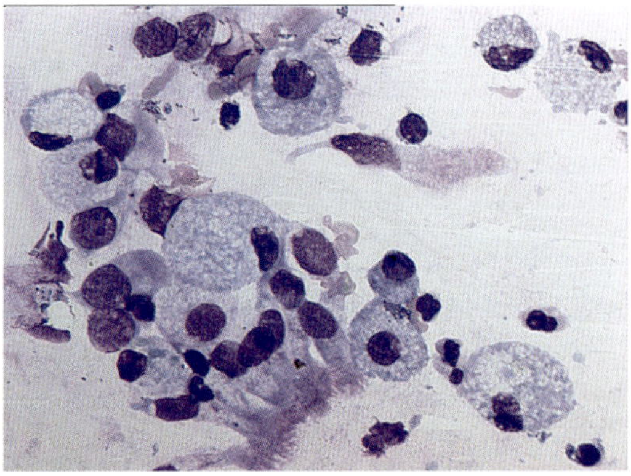

Figure 6.1: Aggregation of storage cells in the lavage fluid.

Blood transfusions

In advanced stages of hypersplenism and hepatic insufficiency, the administration of platelet and erythrocyte concentrates may be necessary. However, the indication for this should be restrictive because transfusions can further exacerbate hypersplenism. In addition, red blood cell concentrates contain large amounts of sphingomyelin. In contrast to Gaucher disease, leukopenia is regularly found in ASMD. Clinically significant granulocytopenias may occur, especially in the setting of viral infections.

Splenectomy

Equivalent to Gaucher disease, complete and partial splenectomies were also performed in the 1970s and 1980s for Niemann-Pick type B disease. Considerations behind this procedure were that the enormous enlargement of the spleen becomes a mechanical obstacle, the theoretical risk of splenic rupture (no case has been described in the literature), and that the storage cells in the spleen consume a significant proportion of dietary calories (Mylla Neto et al. 1983). A counterargument that has been repeatedly listed is the fear of worsening pulmonary involvement. Based on the experience with Gaucher disease, it seems advisable to be very cautious about the indication for splenectomy.

Pregnancy

Female Niemann-Pick type B patients with low disease severity, no significant liver involvement, no bleeding tendency, and no signs of disease progression may well successfully carry a pregnancy to term. The gynecologist and metabolic specialist should monitor the pregnancy as a team. From our own experience, the peripartum bleeding tendency in Niemann-Pick type B disease appears to be less pronounced than in Gaucher disease, as long as no disturbance of liver synthesis capacity is yet present.

Coronary heart disease

Coronary heart disease is a complication of Niemann-Pick type B disease that has received attention in recent years. Since storage cell infiltration of the coronary arteries is assumed to be the causative factor and dyslipidemia (low HDL) plays a minor role, the use of statins to prevent coronary artery disease makes little sense. The therapy (acetylsalicylic acid, bypass surgery, stenting) depends on the cardiological findings. Of course, the other aspects of the disease (e.g., coagulation disorder) must be considered in the cardiological approach.

6.1.2. Causal therapeutic approaches

In individual cases, hematopoietic stem cell transplantations (HSCT) have been successfully performed. However, they are surprisingly not reported in the literature. This may indicate transplant-related problems or insufficient effect on both the central and peripheral nervous systems, but is not supported by facts. HSCT can correct biochemical phenotype and visceral symptoms but has no effect on neurologic involvement. A few months after bone marrow transplantation in a 3-year-old girl with early signs of hepatic failure, the liver was depleted of sphingomyelin and only scattered foam cells were detectable in the bone marrow (Vellodi et al. 1987). More than 15 years later, Ashok Vellodi's group reported on the patient again. At 6 years of age, the first neurological signs were observed. In the meantime, a global encephalopathy with cognitive deficits, peripheral neuropathy and pyramidal tract signs had developed (Victor et al. 2003).

Animal studies on HSCT

HSCT have been extensively studied in animal models. Miranda and co-workers used so-called ASMKO mice for their investigations, in which the *SMPD1* gene was genetically modified to be functionless. With early transplantation and good engraftment, the effect on the reticuloendothelial system was very good. However, even under these ideal conditions, there was no significant effect on the central nervous system (Miranda et al. 1998).

Development of enzyme replacement therapy for Niemann-Pick type B disease

Enzyme replacement therapy has become an important and essential therapeutic principle in metabolic medicine over the past 20 years. Currently, six lysosomal storage disorders can be treated with approved biotechnologically produced enzymes. Additional enzymes are in preclinical and clinical testing, including recombinant sphingomyelinase. The efficacy of enzymes is limited primarily by the fact that intravenously administered enzymes cannot cross the blood-brain barrier. In addition, neurons that have already perished cannot be readily restored.

He and coworkers used sphingomyelinase recombinantly produced in Chinese hamster ovary cells (CHO cells) for their experiments in newborn presymptomatic ASMKO mice. This enzyme can be taken up into cells via the mannose-6-phosphate receptor and reaches the lysosome. In the series of tests, a significant reduction in lipid storage and associated low inflammatory tissue response was found in visceral organs (He et al. 1999). Later, the therapeutic principle was also investigated in older, already diseased mice. The therapeutic effects were clearly apparent, but not as pronounced as with early treatment. Reduction of sphingomyelin storage was most pronounced in the liver, followed by the spleen. Effects on the lungs were less pronounced. This is also reflected in the study result that only 2% of the infused enzyme reaches the lungs. No effect on CNS involvement was seen in either series of experiments (Miranda et al. 2000).

Phase I human clinical trials have been conducted, but the results have not yet been published. The phase I study is an initial investigation into the safety of recombinant sphingomyelinase. Dose-finding studies and dose escalation strategies must follow. It is possible that sphingomyelin metabolism in the liver is much more complex than that of glycolipids (Gaucher disease, Fabry disease). Physicians treating Niemann-Pick type B patients should follow the scientific publications on enzyme replacement therapy in the coming years for the benefit of their patients and maintain contacts with national centers.

6.1.3. Future therapy options

Modified enzyme replacement therapies

The efficacy of enzyme replacement therapy via the mannose-6-phosphate receptor is limited by the inability to cross the blood-brain barrier and the fact that most of the enzyme is directed to the liver. New approaches use alternative receptors to allow the enzyme to cross the blood-brain barrier and be taken up into the cells. Specifically for sphingomyelinase deficiency, cell adhesion molecule-antibody complexes are being studied in the laboratory, the so-called ICAM1 (intercellular adhesion molecule 1) method. A biotechnological enzyme construct consisting of enzyme and receptor binding site of growth hormone was developed on the MPS-VII mouse. Here, uptake into the cell occurs independently of glycosylation via a growth hormone receptor. This technique has not yet been investigated in sphingomyelinase deficiency. Other fusion proteins, consisting of enzyme and antibody against the transferrin binding site at the blood-brain barrier, have now entered clinical trials in Hunter's disease. Years of basic research have aimed to increase the uptake of enzymes across the blood-brain barrier into the brain by targeting various receptors (e.g., insulin and transferrin) located on vascular endothelial cells. Via these receptors, the enzyme, modified as a fusion protein, enters the brain by transcytosis and exerts its effects there. Initial positive results have been reported in preclinical and clinical studies of MPS-I and MPS-II.

Another therapeutic option currently under investigation is the intrathecal application of recombinant sphingomyelinase. Sphingomyelinase deficiency seems to be a very suitable disease for this method because the first neurological symptoms appear later than in infantile courses of other sphingolipidoses (Gaucher disease, Krabbe's disease, Tay-Sachs disease) and the rate of progression is by far not as dramatic. A realistic "therapeutic window" opens up here.

Gene therapy

Various forms of gene therapy were investigated in ASMKO mice. Both *in vivo* and *ex vivo* approaches via cell transplantation were used. Delivery of the *SMPD1* gene into bone marrow cells appears to be most promising using retroviruses. Here, bone marrow must be transplanted after transfection.

In vivo approaches have been primarily investigated using AAV vectors. This vector has also been used to stereotactically deliver the enzyme directly to the CNS. These experiments were associated with some positive results in the mouse model. The enzyme distributed in the brain, significant histological improvements were observed, and the lifespan of the mice normalized.

Despite the promising approaches in animal models, the transition to clinical trials appears exceedingly problematic. Many safety-related questions of genetic engineering still seem unresolved, making it impossible to give a prognosis. This is also against the background that no unfulfillable expectations and hopes should be raised in patients.

References

He X, et al. 1999. Characterization of human acid sphingomyelinase purified from the media of overexpressing Chinese hamster ovary cells. Biochim Biophys Acta 1432 (2): 251-64

Miranda SR, et al. 1998. Biochemical, pathological, and clinical response to transplantation of normal bone marrow cells into acid sphingomyelinase-deficient mice. Transplantation 65(7): 884-92

Miranda SR, et al. 2000. Infusion of recombinant human acid sphingomyelinase into niemann-pick disease mice leads to visceral, but not neurological, correction of the pathophysiology. FASEB J 14(13): 1988-95

Mylla Neto G, et al. 1983. Niemann-Pick disease in adult: report of a case surgically treated. Rev Hosp Clin Fac Med Sao Paulo 38(2): 83-5

Nicholson AG, et al. 2002. Successful treatment of endogenous lipoid pneumonia due to Niemann-Pick Type B disease with whole-lung lavage. Am J Respir Crit Care Med 165(1): 128-31

Vellodi A, et al. 1987. Treatment of Niemann-Pick disease type B by allogeneic bone marrow transplantation. Br Med J (Clin Res Ed) 295(6610): 1375-6

Victor S, et al. 2003. Niemann-Pick disease: sixteen-year follow-up of allogeneic bone marrow transplantation in a type B variant. J Inherit Metab Dis 26(8): 775-85

6.2. Management and treatment of Niemann-Pick type C disease

When it was discovered in the 1980s that lysosomal storage of cholesterol significantly characterizes the pathobiology of NPC, it was reasonable to conclude that cholesterol-lowering drugs might also positively influence the course of NPC. Patterson and coworkers at the National Institutes of Health (NIH) studied the effects of colestyramine, lovastatin, nicotinic acid and dimethyl sulfoxide in 25 patients. Except for dimethyl sulfoxide, all drugs lowered plasma and liver cholesterol levels, but neurologic symptoms, once again, were unaffected (Patterson et al. 1993).

It took more than 10 years for a new drug, miglustat, to enter clinical trials in NPC. Miglustat has been approved for the treatment of Gaucher type 1 disease of mild or moderate severity for almost 10 years in cases where enzyme replacement therapy is not an option (Cox et al. 2003).

Since January 2009, miglustat has also been available for the treatment of Niemann-Pick type C disease. For the first time, neurological symptoms of a lysosomal disease can thus be treated not only symptomatically. The drug intervenes in the neuropathological metabolism of the disease. A whole series of other substances are currently being investigated in preclinical studies for their potential effect on NPC (Wraith et al. 2009).

Until 2009, at best supportive therapies were available to improve patients' quality of life and alleviate suffering. Supportive therapies, such as those for spasticity, aspiration and pain, require high standards of quality medical care, especially in the late stages of the disease. Non-NPC-specific drugs are available to treat dystonia, cataplexy and epilepsy.

In 2018, under the umbrella of the International Niemann-Pick Disease Alliance, a network of scientists, led by Geberhiwot, published guidelines on current diagnosis, treatment and monitoring of patients with NPC. This document presents general guidelines that the authors believe can inform providers and physicians about the needs of patients with NPC to ensure equitable and improved care.

International Niemann-Pick Disease Registry (INPDR)

INPDR is a not-for-profit, registered company in the United Kingdom. It provides an opportunity to expand knowledge and understanding of Niemann-Pick disease by reaching patients around the world and using high-quality data. It realizes a global collaboration between patient associations, clinicians and scientists working together for the benefit of patients and their families everywhere.

The registry includes and is supported by a network of 16 NPD patient support groups and charities in 15 different countries. In addition, INPDR is supported by professional partners involved in the care of patients with all types of Niemann-Pick disease (ASMD and NPC).

The goal of the INPDR is to develop and maintain a unique patient-managed database that supports research and therapy development and improves the care and treatment of patients with Niemann-Pick disease through global collaboration. This will be achieved by:

- continued use of data to improve the broader understanding of Niemann-Pick disease
- support and facilitate rigorous research and therapy development
- promote earlier diagnosis and equitable access to diagnostic testing
- establish the INPDR as a collaborative initiative much needed by patients and professionals alike.

There is a legitimate hope that this groundbreaking initiative will inspire further global collaboration between patient groups, clinicians, scientists, researchers and pharmaceutical companies, all working together to improve care and treatment options for patients with Niemann-Pick disease worldwide.

TheEuropean Medicines Agency (EMA) guidelines aimed at raising standards for long-term safety studies of drugs (pharmacovigilance) encourage the use of independent disease-specific patient registries. INPDR is currently working with a number of companies that are considering using the registry to conduct long-term safety studies or in development of new therapies.

The pharmaceutical companies with whom we cooperate do not have access to patient-level data, and all data requests we receive are carefully reviewed by the Scientific Advisory Committee (SAC). Collaboration with the industry helps to improve their research and studies, as well as secure resources to support the ongoing work of INPDR.

6.2.1. Miglustat

The biochemical substance N-butyl-deoxynojirimycin (NB-DNJ) was given the name miglustat in pharmacology. As an iminosugar, miglustat is a so-called small-molecule (☞ Figure 6.2).

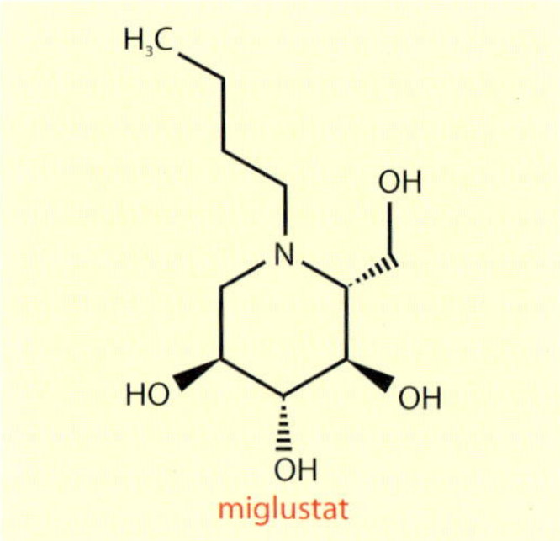

Figure 6.2: Structural formula of miglustat.

NB-DNJ was first investigated in HIV research in the 1990s (Fischer et al. 1996). However, it was shown to have only a minor effect on retroviruses. The effect of miglustat on the key enzyme of ganglioside synthesis, glucosylceramide synthase (GCS), only came into focus later in the 1990s (Platt et al. 2001). Competitive inhibition of GCS inhibits the synthesis of glucosylceramide – the storage product of Gaucher disease. Glucosylceramide is the basic element of the neurotoxic glucosylceramides GM3- and GM2-ganglioside and lactosylceramide. The metabolism of sphingomyelin remains unaffected. This mechanism of action promised for the first time that a drug might be able to break the lipid transport congestion in neuronal cells and thus intervene directly in neuropathological processes. A second mechanism of action in neuronal cells has been hypothesized to be the correction of intracellular calcium hemostasis by lowering glucosylceramide concentrations (Lloyd-Evans et al. 2003). Pioneering work towards clinical trials has now been carried out in animal models by the research group led by Steve Walkley. In both the mouse model and the cat model, it was shown that neurological symptoms commence later and that survival time was prolonged by about 20% (Zervas et al. 2001). Another prerequisite for a positive effect of miglustat in humans is that the substance must be able to cross the human blood-brain barrier. Studies in the rat animal model suggested this is likely (Treiber et al. 2007).

Safety and efficacy of miglustat was studied in 29 patients (adolescents and young adults older than 12 years) and 12 children younger than 12 years. While all patients in the pediatric study received verum, the study with patients older than 12 years was controlled and randomized 2:1 versus standard care. In addition, 5-year follow-up data from this cohort on treatment with miglustat have been published. A significant improvement in saccade velocity (HSEM-alpha) in the verum group versus standard treatment was observed at 12 months. Sustained stabilization was seen after 24 months. Further improvements in individual cases were seen in swallowing, walking ability and cognition. In patients treated with miglustat for more than 12 months, stabilization was seen in three-quarters of patients. Stabilization in this setting was defined as at least consistent findings of the primary and secondary study endpoints (HSEM-alpha, swallowing, walking ability, cognition). Further information on the efficacy and safety of miglustat emerged from a retrospective multicenter observational study in 66 predominantly pediatric NPC patients followed with the modified Itturiaga disease-specific NPC score. The majority of patients showed a stable NPC score that remained unchanged over time. Improvements in NPC score were seen primarily in patients with late manifestation of NPC.

The studies in NPC patients showed a comparable side effect profile compared to previous studies. In the foreground are gastrointestinal side effects such as diarrhea, flatulence and weight loss, which still affect about 50% of patients. The gastrointestinal side effects mostly regress after an initial phase and can be well managed with dietary changes (Belmatoug et al. 2011). In the past, the gastrointestinal side effects were thought to be most likely caused by induced lactose intolerance. Preliminary evidence is now emerging that a competitive inhibition of intestinal disaccharidases is the cause. Tremor is also regularly seen, which is reversible on discontinuation or dose reduction.

The recommended dosage in NPC patients older than 12 years is 3 × 200 mg. In children younger than 12 years, the dosage must be adjusted according to the body surface area. In infants with infantile and rapidly progressing manifestations and in patients with end-stage disease, it should be considered, in accordance with international recommendations, that the expected therapeutic success, which may be small at best, does not outweigh the side effects (Wraith et al. 2009).

In summary, miglustat can modify but not cure neurologic symptoms in NPC. Patients with late manifestation in adolescence and adulthood respond best to therapy. Gastrointestinal side effects are common but mostly well managed. Miglustat has no effect on visceral symptoms of the disease.

6.2.2. Bone marrow and liver transplantations

Some experimental therapy trials with bone marrow and combined bone marrow and liver transplantation, as well as studies in animal models, demonstrate that transplantation is ineffective in NPC1 disease. In individual cases, liver transplantation has been performed in children with cholestatic liver failure in ignorance of the diagnosis of NPC without favorably affecting the neuropathic course of the disease. The metabolic defect of a complex transmembrane protein probably cannot be corrected in principle by transplantation.

NPC2 disease must be assessed differently. Since the NPC2 protein is a soluble lysosomal glycoprotein, correction with hematopoietic stem cell transplantation is conceivable, on a par with other lysosomal enzyme defects. A first publication on hematopoietic stem cell transplantation appeared in 2010, but this paper did not yet report on the long-term outcome. Therefore, this therapy must still be considered experimental. Furthermore, it has to be considered that infants with NPC2 are mostly in such a poor general condition that a transplantation is not feasible.

6.2.3. Treatment of extrapyramidal symptoms, spasticity, cataplexy and epilepsy

Dystonia and tremor are regularly observed as extrapyramidal symptoms in NPC. When symptoms are disabling, anticholinergics are most likely indicated. The therapeutic response is mostly satisfactory, but side effects must be considered. For movement disorders, adjunctive physiotherapy is indicated.

Cataplexies should be treated according to the Narcolepsy Guideline of the German Society of Neurology. Psychostimulants, sodium oxybate and antidepressants are used. Clomipramine and sodium oxybate (covered by the Narcotics Act [BtMG] in Germany) are thought to have a good effect on cataplexy. Other antidepressants or MAO inhibitors and psychostimulants may also be effective. In individual cases, the association of cataplexy and focal seizures may be a problem and complicate therapy.

In the advanced course, progressive spasticity can significantly reduce the patient's quality of life. Systemically effective drugs such as baclofen often have unacceptable side effects. Local therapies with botulinum toxin, for example in the case of painful subluxation of the hip, can be used very effectively here.

Epileptic seizures, mostly complex-focal, are observed in 30-50% of NPC patients. The choice of anticonvulsant is also guided by the semiology: Lamotrigine or oxcarbazepine for more focal seizures, valproate for primarily generalized seizures. Occasionally, combination therapies become necessary. Satisfactory seizure control is usually achievable. Lamotrigine and valproate have the advantage of being affect-stabilizing. In contrast, levetiracetam can cause significant mood swings and agitated behavior in NPC patients and should only be used under strict observation and consideration.

6.2.4. Substances in preclinical and experimental studies

In experiments with cells exhibiting NPC pathology, overexpression of the GTPase Rab9 leads to restoration of pathological lipid transport. This is a promising observation and should be further investigated in NPC animal models. Perhaps, even if no therapeutic option emerges, at least the regulation of intracellular lipid transport can be better understood.

Neurosteroids influence neuronal cell growth and differentiation and the action of neurotransmitters and their receptors. Experiments with the neurosteroid pregnanolone showed an astonishing response after a single administration shortly after birth. However, further studies showed that the effective agent here is not pregnanolone but the solvent beta-cyclodextrin. Beta-cyclodextrin in high doses leads to a significant reduction in lipid storage in both the liver and brain of the NPC mouse. The lifespan of the animals doubled.

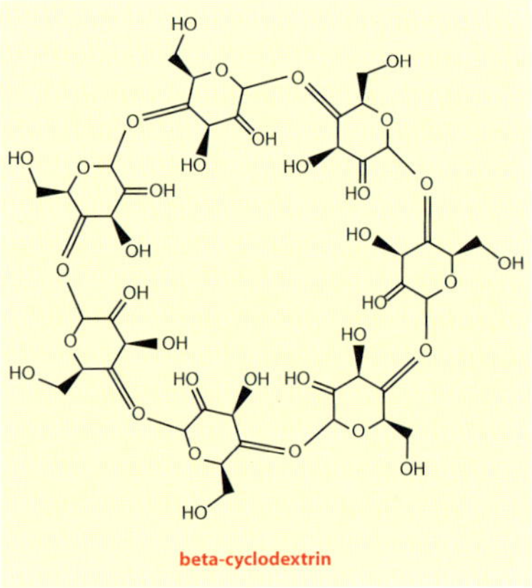

Figure 6.3: Structural formula of beta-cyclodextrin.

Of course, it is not possible to transfer these results to humans without further investigation. Side effects have to be taken into account that cannot be observed in the animal model. In addition, it must be considered that the animals were treated a few weeks after birth before the onset of neurological symptoms.

Further substances that show some effect in animal models are imitanib, curcumin and non-steroidal anti-inflammatory drugs. These certainly do not have the potential to become established as monotherapy, but in combination with miglustat or even beta-cyclodextrin, an additional benefit can be hoped for. Further preclinical studies are needed to form a definitive opinion.

Cyclodextrin is currently being investigated as an intravenous application in clinical trials. The studies on intrathecal administration were stopped after initial positive results in phase III clinical trials (☞ www.clinicaltrials.gov).

References

Belmatoug N, Burlina A, Giraldo P, Hendriksz CJ, Kuter DJ, et al. 2011. Gastrointestinal disturbances and their management in miglustat-treated patients. J Inherit Metab Dis 34: 991-1001

Cox TM, Aerts JM, Andria G, Beck M, Belmatoug N, et al. 2003. The role of the iminosugar N-butyldeoxynojirimycin (miglustat) in the management of type I (non-neuronopathic) Gaucher disease: a position statement. J Inherit Metab Dis 26: 513-26

Fischer PB, Karlsson GB, Butters TD, Dwek RA, Platt FM. 1996. N-butyldeoxynojirimycin-mediated inhibition of human immunodeficiency virus entry correlates with changes in antibody recognition of the V1/V2 region of gp120. J Virol 70: 7143-52

Lloyd-Evans E, Pelled D, Riebeling C, Bodennec J, de-Morgan A, et al. 2003. Glucosylceramide and glucosylsphingosine modulate calcium mobilization from brain microsomes via different mechanisms. J Biol Chem 278: 23594-9

Patterson MC, Di Bisceglie AM, Higgins JJ, Abel RB, Schiffmann R, et al. 1993. The effect of cholesterol-lowering agents on hepatic and plasma cholesterol in Niemann-Pick disease type C. Neurology 43: 61-4

Platt FM, Jeyakumar M, Andersson U, Priestman DA, Dwek RA, et al. 2001. Inhibition of substrate synthesis as a strategy for glycolipid lysosomal storage disease therapy. J Inherit Metab Dis 24: 275-90

Treiber A, Morand O, Clozel M. 2007. The pharmacokinetics and tissue distribution of the glucosylceramide synthase inhibitor miglustat in the rat. Xenobiotica; the fate of foreign compounds in biological systems 37: 298-314

Wraith JE, Baumgartner MR, Bembi B, Covanis A, Levade T, et al. 2009. Recommendations on the diagnosis and management of Niemann-Pick disease type C. Mol Genet Metab 98: 152-65

Zervas M, Somers KL, Thrall MA, Walkley SU. 2001. Critical role for glycosphingolipids in Niemann-Pick disease type C. Curr Biol 11: 1283-7

Index